SOARING IN YOUR FAITH AND FITNESS

Inviting God on the Journey

SOARING IN YOUR FAITH AND FITNESS

Inviting God on the Journey

APRIL GRIFFITH

Front Cover Photography: Hannah Capps

ACKNOWLEDGEMENTS

First, to my Lord and Savior Jesus Christ. Thank you for keeping me and getting me this far. Everything I am and everything I've learned is because of you and Your great mercy!

To my Pastor and Assistant Pastor/First Lady, thank you for the Word you have taught me over the years that prayerfully flood these pages and impact many lives.

To my parents, thank you for everything you have done for me and instilled in me over the years through the good and hard times. You continue to support me in everything I do even until this day and I love you immensely for it.

I also dedicate this book to the memory of my Granny and Auntie Renee, I miss you so much and wish you were here to see this day. Auntie, you always encouraged me and told me I was perfect. And now I hope to inspire others to see their perfection too.

TABLE OF CONTENTS

INTRODUCTION

Beloved, welcome!

I'm so delighted and honored that you are holding this book in your hands. I didn't write this book because I'm a super athlete, because I get it right every time or because I may be the best fitness coach in the world, or even the United States. Okay, maybe not even in my state or city, but I am really passionate about seeing believers excel in their health and wellness by relying on their faith and inviting God on the journey.

This book is not about focusing on your past, not about what you can't do or even what you might find difficult to do. It was written as an encouragement for you, the person reading this book right now to believe, "with God, all things are possible" (Matthew 19:26).

We know this scripture all too well, in addition to another favorite "I can do all things through Christ who strengthens me." (Philippians 4:13). However, we don't really seem to incorporate or stand on these scriptures when it comes to our health, wellness and definitely not our fitness. I hear my clients say all the time "I can't do that" without even trying. At that moment, Philippians 4:13 is not at the forefront of their minds unfortunately.

This book is really about coupling those concepts with your fitness journey, as you do in other areas of your life like finances, family and even your job. Your health is no different and is just as important as those other areas.

I remember hearing a presenter give a statistic that "more people die from obesity than hunger." I was both alarmed and angered. This set me on a mission. I was determined to help everyone possible, avoid falling into the pitfalls of obesity. I am so passionate about this, because I saw a gap in the Body of Christ. Not only were many of us unhealthy, but we were not seeing how to solve the problem through our faith and the Word of God.

For some reason, health and wellness are not discussed much. For some reason, we don't talk about glorifying God in our bodies. For some reason, we breeze over scriptures where God says to glorify Him in our bodies—"Or do you not know that your body is the temple of the Holy Spirit who is in you, whom you have from God, and you are not your own? For you were bought at a price; therefore glorify God in your body and in your spirit, which are God's." (1 Corinthians 6:19-20).

Now, I know that in this text Paul was alluding to sexual sin and immorality. However, do you hear the heart about us glorifying God? If you don't get anything else except "you are not your own," that should put some perspective on how you should treat your body. For some reason, we lean on the healing prayer line rather than being proactive and even breaking the curse. Nothing wrong with the healing prayer line! I believe in healing and the laying on of hands. Some things require that. Others require us to be good stewards.

The pages that follow will be less of a prescription of the kind of fitness you should do, and more of a template for exercising your faith muscle to be successful in your fitness journey. The principles can be applied to any area of life and many times are. Because they are so often forgotten in this area, I wanted to connect the dots.

You will find key lessons to ponder in every chapter. I encourage you to ask God for further revelation to apply these lessons practically to your life and journey.

You will also find that there are scripture references included for you to confess daily, or multiple times per day, until you see evidence of the symptom you are applying the scripture to leave, just like a medical prescription. Some call these affirmations. As long as you are affirming what the Word says about you, I'm okay with that!

You may need to go back and review the scriptures after finishing the chapter, because the enemy of your soul will continue to come after you, time and time again in these areas, to steal what you have put in. John 10:10 says, "The thief comes to steal kill and destroy." It's okay to head immediately to the next chapter after confessing the scriptures at the end. However, know that these are not just nice to have or to be lightly glanced over. These are mighty weapons, carefully selected for you to put in your arsenal to actually use every time the enemy shows his ugly face.

Lastly, you will find a prayer to the Father's heart that you can pray. I would also encourage you to add your own words and speak directly to your Heavenly Father. He cares and He is listening. It is also good to take a little time to be quiet and still after your prayer to see if He whispers anything back into your ear. It may or may not happen at this time, but it is my heart and goal to always have a listening ear for whenever He may drop an important instruction, sweet note or even a joke. My point here is to be quick to listen and act on whatever He says.

I pray this book blesses you, encourages you and stirs you in your faith. May you soar in every aspect of your life, including your fitness journey.

CHAPTER ONE

MAKING THE DECISION

The First Step

It was a beautiful summer day on a beautiful campus near the lake. We were all gathered in a room that seemed to be the basement, but it was much nicer than an average run-of-the-mill basement at the bottom of a building. I remember walking down the steps being a little nervous but everyone I encountered greeted me with a huge smile. That eased my nervousness a little.

The overwhelming joy on everyone's face seemed genuine enough but at the same time, a little strange. And definitely different from what I was used to! Rows of chairs filled the space with an aisle separating the right from the left side of the room. It wasn't completely packed, but those who were there definitely wanted to be there. Those smiles communicated that clearly, which again was a little different for me.

Everything seemed to move along smoothly that night - nothing weird. And then it happened, the big ask came at the end and nearly knocked me over! Not like a ton of bricks, but more like a soft, light-weight feather, gentle and full of love, from this young college-aged guy in jeans and a polo. Is this why they brought me here? Was this the plan all along? Was I set up? Each of these questions quickly rushed through my head.

But amidst all the questions flooding my brain, the kind, gentle voice broke through and said, "If Jesus were to return tonight, would you go with Him?" "Wait! What?" I thought in my head, "Jesus return? Oh, yes, I have heard that He is coming back, but is that what He meant? Tonight? Would I? Of course, no one knows the day or hour but if that hour were now, would I go with Him? Would He take me with Him?" I wasn't sure. I didn't know! His next set of instructions was so simple that I finally calmed my brain down and was confident I had to do it. I raised my hand and made a decision that night to accept Jesus, the Christ, into my heart and life as Lord and Savior - and I haven't looked back.

This was the most important decision I could have and will ever make in life. Likewise, for anyone else who accepts Christ! That means there are other decisions to be made. We make decisions every day, multiple times a day. And each of those decisions shapes our experiences. So, our decisions have consequences, good or bad, and our decisions dictate what we truly believe. Now this isn't scriptural but as my grandma would say, "If you hang around dogs, you will get fleas." You probably see where I'm going here. The pages that follow will be focused on fitness and wellness from a biblical perspective.

Since you are reading this book, chances are you have made a decision to take control of your health and wellness and are probably starting a journey to get your fitness together. If not, you may still be on the "I know I need to do something" boat, but maybe you haven't fully made the decision. If that's you, stick around until the end and let's see if any of this helped you. The third category could be you have been on the journey for some time but know it's time to go higher, so soaring caught your attention. Or perhaps there is a fourth category: You get the health and wellness, the fitness part, however you've never considered inviting God on the journey and relying on your faith. Until now, you have been relying on yourself, and maybe even what the world has told you. If that is the case, perfect - stick around. This can encourage you too!

Whether you have made the decision or are very close to making the decision to transform into a healthier, more whole you, my prayer is you realize, by the end of this book, the benefits and wisdom in including your faith in this process and asking God to join you along the journey! Saying yes in this area means we are well on our way! (Woo Hoo!) Making this decision suggests that you have discovered your "why" or at least in my opinion, the most important part of your "why." You may be wondering, "What is a 'why', April?"

The Why?

Well, I'm glad you asked me! And it's not just because "I said so," like you may have heard your mom say growing up, lol. Well, maybe a little, but I only said so for your benefit. Do you remember the commercial of the little girl continuously asking her dad, "Why? Why? Why?" Every time he answered her question, she asked another "why" to that answer. I can hear it so clearly in my head as I write, which is hilarious, but don't worry, it's not going to be one of those "why" conversations. This is a way to drill down on why you are doing what you are doing, but I will spare you that conversation for now.

In its simplest explanation, your "why" may be summed up in the people, places and things that make you realize *why* you have made the decision or need to make the decision to go on this journey and turn a new page to a new you. Why you're moving forward in a new direction to take control of your health and wellness; and why you will be a good steward of what God has entrusted to you! Why you will be committed and faithful on this journey going forward. Afterall, faithfulness is necessary in stewardship (1 Corinthians 4:2).

In addition to faithfulness, Jesus also taught us to be wise stewards: "And the Lord said, 'Who then is that faithful and wise steward, whom his master will make ruler over his household, to give them their portion of food in due season?'" (Luke 12:42); and "He who is faithful in what is least is faithful also in much; and he who is unjust in what is least is unjust also in much." (Luke 16:10). As we can see, the Bible talks a lot about stewardship and this is just scratching the surface. In my opinion this "why", focusing on His plan for your life, including salvation and you being a good steward has to be your number one "why"!

If I asked you if God loves you, you would probably tell me "yes." I could ask you how you know and you may go back to the old Sunday School song "Yes, Jesus loves me because the Bible tells me so." But do you really believe this? I always tell people their actions will always follow their beliefs. When you know God loves you so much and loves to be included, and even more so, invited into every one of your decisions, would you believe me? Would you do it? This includes how He wants to help you navigate a healthy and active lifestyle?

Inviting Him in makes the journey that much more exciting and attainable. You are no longer leaning on your own understanding (Proverbs 3:4). You are seeking Him for direction, praying to Him for understanding, asking Him for wisdom. To prevent you making this another fad or diet that you won't keep, you are going to Him when things get rough and you want to quit.

You are celebrating the success with Him when goals and milestones are met. You are not only saying it, but actually demonstrating, that Him being there is important, that His help is critical and necessary for you to make this kingdom shift. You need Holy Spirit, who lives inside of you, to do His job, to be your teacher and guide in this area of your life just as you do for your finances, children, career and so on, as 1 John 4:4 teaches: "You are of God, little children, and have overcome them, because He who is in you is greater than he who is in the world."

The price Christ paid for you through salvation - and salvation extends beyond just going to heaven - proves that He is committed to you in every way. Now it's time for you to be committed to you as well! The Word of God declares, that "You are fearfully and wonderfully made" (Psalm 139:14), "You have been bought with a price" (1Corthians 6:19). That alone is reason enough for your "why!" But if you need more "whys," consider your family, spouse, children, parents, siblings, friends, your clients, your church. They all need you too. I believe God honors your obedience in this decision to change and live your best, healthiest life for Him and in Him.

Your "whys" need you to operate in optimal health. It hurts them to see you on tons of medication, getting negative reports from the doctor and barely being able to breathe when you walk. This is especially hurtful in communities with food deserts and higher health risks. We have to change something. Your "why" needs you, we need you, the world needs you!

One of the most challenging parts about my mom and my relationship, if I can be completely transparent, is her health. We have these conversations all the time. And while I am praying for her health daily, it pains me and frustrates me when she can't walk a block without being short of breath or has to take a seat every couple of steps. Now, I will also be honest and say that another level of patience and compassion needs to be developed in me in this area. However, I don't believe this is God's best for her. As I write this book, I'm still praying and believing God for her breakthrough. I want her to realize her "why" and make some lasting changes as I'm suggesting with you. She has lost some weight so we are on our way.

Now let me ask you, are your kids or spouse or siblings missing out on you? Are they frustrated by continuous hospital visits or astronomical prescription bills? Is there an absence of quality time walking along a trail, throwing a ball around the yard or taking a bike ride through the neighborhood because of your health? Are you showing up for them in your health like you are with providing a roof over their head? Food for thought! So, when you feel like giving up, remember these people, places and things and keep going. Remember your "why." This journey is about God, you and those counting on you!

If you are saying, or thinking you don't even have a "why", I challenge you. Everyone has a "why." Even if you don't have family or anyone you are close to, there are people you are meant to reach in this world, who need you to be functioning in the best health possible. Again, remember the first "why," - Christ and the price He paid for you to live, and live more abundantly (John

10:10). If for Christ alone, it's worth the continuous push. So, let's start there!

If you need other "whys," consider diseases that plague us, like high blood pressure, diabetes, cardiovascular disease, cholesterol, and so on. Hypertension is considered the silent killer. Research has shown that even walking reduces chances of cardiovascular disease, according to the American Heart Association (www.heart.org). Now let's get moving! He and all of heaven are pulling for you, so that's the best "why" ever! I also encourage people to keep visuals around you at all times - pictures, scriptures, anything that reminds you and points you back to your goal.

Because there will be times when you will want to quit and give up (which we will talk about in a later chapter), your "whys" have to bring you back to a state of victory and determination. There will certainly be ups and downs. The enemy will be constantly in your ear, but go back to your "why", at these times. It will make things easier; and you can cast every one of those thoughts down, bring them captive to the obedience of Christ (Ephesians 6). The road won't necessarily be easy, but using this weapon will make it easier. If it were easy, everyone would be doing it! It takes hard work, determination and sacrifice to win this faith and fitness race.

There will be times when you may even wonder if God is on your side, if He is still there. If you feel like that, it means the enemy is definitely resisting you because he knows the great breakthrough God has for you. I would even go so far as to say you are gaining ground! If there is anything the enemy can do to stop you, he will, including telling you countless lies like "It's not working; you can't do this; it's too hard for you; you are wasting your time." If you hear anything remotely similar to one of those scripts, reject it immediately.

Don't quit! Go back to your "whys" and keep pushing! Knowing your "why" is critical in the decision-making phase. Your "why" keeps you going when no one supports you, when you feel like giving up, and when you don't see any change. I heard a coach say, "It's not how your start, it's how you finish. You are either moving forward or moving backward, there is no in-between." No progress is equivalent to retreating, because when you remain still and stagnant, you are not gaining the ground you should be gaining.

<u>Repent and Turn</u>

The other necessary part of the decision-making phase is repentance. Just as the decision to receive Jesus into my heart and life, I had to make the decision to repent of my sin. I had to acknowledge I was a sinner; I needed a Savior and Christ died for my redemption. I needed to ask Him to come in and clean me. In the same way, we need to repent for where we haven't treated our bodies as the temples of the Living God. We need to ask God to forgive us where we have allowed diseases to live in our bodies because of our negligence; where we have lived sedentary lives that have not allowed us to live in His fullness and perform all the work He has called us to do; where we have allowed issues of the past to bring us into a place of feeling unworthy, emotional eating, disordered eating and not living in the richness of what He initially created us to live in.

Please, please, please don't take this the wrong way and send me hate mail saying I'm being insensitive. I know all the above issues are real and serious and people are hurting as a result, so please hear my heart. This isn't about condemnation, it is about recognizing our part and owning it if we have done anything, and repenting for that. It's not about shame.

The enemy wants to shame us, but the Holy Spirt convicts us if we allow Him to. Embracing that conviction is where we begin to see change. Once we repent, it is under the blood of Jesus, not to be remembered any more by you, especially because He doesn't. This is about a clean slate, a new beginning, a fresh start. The old ways and behaviors are gone, by faith through repentance, and all things have become new.

One translation of the word repentance is to turn. This is the time to turn - turn from old habits, unhealthy limiting belief systems, sedentary lifestyles, self-sabotaging behaviors and so on. It's time! The Bible calls us to repent. It's not anything to be ashamed of or shy away from. It actually helps us in drawing closer to God - "Repent therefore and be converted, that your sins may be blotted out, so that times of refreshing may come from the presence of the Lord." (Acts 3:19).

Repentance is not a bad thing. I know it seems like an ugly word, has a bad reputation, but it is so necessary for us to walk closely with Christ. And if there were ever a time that we need to walk closely with God, it's now and it's in our health.

Let's Talk Goals

After repentance comes time to set some goals. Reasonable, Actionable Goals (RAG). These are similar to the SMART goals you may have learned about in the workplace or at school. It's okay to have a big dream or vision which we will talk about more a little later, but tangible goals on how we will get there are very important! Equally important is writing them down, making them real and working towards them to keep yourself accountable. This takes personal responsibility. I'm sure you have heard that a goal not written down is just a nice idea. We need to make these goals so real to us that no one can convince us not to have them. Declaring and decreeing a thing like the Bible talks about is the next piece we will talk about — "You will also declare a thing, And it will be established for you; So light will shine on your ways." (Job 22:28).

One thing with goals. Many people think goals have to be huge, but they don't. It's perfectly fine to have large goals that will blow your mind when you see them come to pass, but it's also perfectly fine to have small goals, medium goals and everything in between. What I want you to remember is starting off small is okay. It is important for you to celebrate even the small accomplishments. Celebrate every one every time! This will let you know it's achievable and spur you on to the next goal, so you are more likely to crush it as well.

Sometimes we bite off more than we can chew, so to speak, which can lead to overwhelm and discouragement if the original goal is not met. This doesn't mean we can't bounce back, but it does mean it is okay to start small working our way towards larger goals and even consult with God on a RAG even before we set them. Remember, we invited Him in on this journey, so He's present, ready to assist with your goals too! And just a quick PSA (public service announcement, not the medical term, hahaha) for all who are reading and listening - everyone starts at zero. Your goal is to not stay there! Do not despise the days of small beginnings. Keep at it. You will get there!

For example, if you started off doing five pushups, and your goal is to be able to do twenty, once you get to twenty it's going to be amazing. However, I caution you not to get discouraged if it takes longer to get to twenty than you may have anticipated. That is why we set reasonable actionable goals (RAGs) and more importantly why we invited God on this journey. Perhaps you wanted to hit twenty by week three and it didn't happen. Keep going, even if it takes you until week seven. Continue to believe that you can do all things through Christ who strengthens you

(Philippians 4:13). Stop at nothing until you hit the twenty pushups. 'All things' means exactly that, ALL things! You've got this!

That brings me to attaching time frames with goals. It's always good to put a date or timeframe next to your goal. This heightens your accountability and gives you something tangible to measure and work towards. If you don't hit the timeframe the first time, that's okay. Recalibrate and set another timeframe or date as in the example above. It may have been that the first one was not reasonable, or it may be that you have to go harder to get there. In the pushup example, you may need more focus on your upper body, and that's okay. Goals with timeframes let you know exactly where you are! And as long as you get there, that's the ultimate goal. Quitting cannot be an option!

Getting Started

But where do I begin?" you may ask. My simple response is just get started and get moving. Walking is probably one of the easiest ways to get moving. It's free and doesn't require any equipment. Don't let not knowing where to start delay you. Delayed progress isn't actually progress at all. I have even heard it said "Delay is the enemy of wealth." Now, correlate wealth and health—your health is your wealth. Therefore, you can't afford to delay any longer.

One school of thought is that unsuccessful people make delayed decisions but that's not you, right? It doesn't take a major fitness overhaul to start moving. Based upon your current physical activity level, take realistic steps from there. If you have not performed any exercise in months, perhaps starting with a walk simple is ideal. Time your walk on the first outing and then continue to improve on that time with the next walk and the next walk. As you continue to grow, keep beating your time and challenging yourself. Soon you will be jogging and even running!

If you have recently performed some type of physical activity, you might find a gym or trainer like me to work with and challenge you, or you may find a video on YouTube. There are a ton of resources available to you. The point here is not to overthink it and let that paralyze you. That's called fear, my friend. And we won't let fear stop us. When we invite God in, His perfect love casts out all fear. "There is no fear in love; but perfect love casts out fear, because fear involves torment. But he who fears has not been made perfect in love." (1 John 4:18).

I do believe some people may need more structure and accountability to be to remain focused. That is where a program or a coach may be the right choice. Each of our programs at Kingdom Power Living is based upon two fundamental concepts—Consistency and Accountability, built upon a solid foundation of faith. Now, that makes for a terrific trio!

<u>Being Committed</u>

After goals and getting started, commitment is key! Have you ever heard that saying "Commitment is key"? Well, it's true. Ask yourself who and what are you committed to. Be brutally honest. If it doesn't start with God, followed by you and/or your spouse, children if you have them, and so on, it's time to get committed! You have to be committed to the process and to yourself! There is unfortunately no way around it. You know where you haven't been committed to YOU up until this point, but that's why you are reading this book. That's why we are having this conversation. And I'm so glad we are. But now is the time! If not now, then when?

You have to be your biggest cheerleader, your number one fan. Even if no one else is in your corner, including a spouse if applicable, your mom or your best friend, it doesn't matter. God is committed to you, so you must be committed to Him as well as to the temple He has entrusted to you. No more cutting corners, no more putting off today what you say you will do tomorrow and then don't! No more mediocracy, no more lukewarmness, no more wishing and not going after it, no more excuses. No more, no more, no more!!! It's game time and commitment is key! So, say it after me "Yes, I will commit. I will commit to God. I will commit to me. I will commit to my health and wellness. I will commit to this process." Let's go!

This commitment means not giving up, eating right, getting your workouts in, saying "no" when it's not good for your body and your spirit. You are committing to not making excuses, committed to your goals, committed to being serious about this lifestyle change. Even being committed when others around you are doing the contrary.

Now this one might be a little difficult but you have to stick to it! The reward is far greater than the momentary struggle, I promise! Even Paul talked about controlling his body. "But I discipline my body and bring it into subjection, lest, when I have preached to others, I myself should become disqualified." (1 Corinthians 9:27).

Become comfortable with saying no to others when it doesn't align with your faith and fitness journey. Be comfortable with being labeled the healthy person; become comfortable with people saying she doesn't eat that or do this. That is okay. That is part of leadership. Standing out in the midst of the crowd is part of leadership. Think about Daniel when he purposed in his heart not to eat the king's delicacies. That was commitment!

This will require you to pay a price. Nothing is free except for salvation. Every day, you have to count the cost and determine if you are going to pay the price to stay healthy and whole. It will not be easy, but no one can take it from you. You can only give it away. Make the choice not to. There is a reason why the road less traveled is called so. Not everyone is committed. That too should drive you. Knowing you are doing things others haven't done and getting the reward others won't get until they too make a decision is a recipe for success.

Commitment also means living in what I like to call the "no excuse zone." There is a difference between reasons and excuses, the biggest difference being personal responsibility and accountability. Excuses usually lean towards justification, pointing the finger, passing the blame. "I couldn't workout this morning because of this or that." A reason says, "The in-laws came over unexpectedly and I got distracted from getting my workout in this morning." See the difference? One accepts the fact that "you" made the decision not to work out, regardless of the unexpected external occurrences.

Yes, there will be external circumstances that distract you and throw you off your game or off your routine. There aren't always ideal or perfect situations. And no one is perfect. God isn't looking for that. When the Bible talks about being perfect it's talking about maturity. You own the situation and figure out what's the pivot plan. Monkey wrenches get thrown at the best of us. Even the most disciplined athlete's plans get twisted and thrown off every once in a while, but it doesn't stop them and it doesn't become a pattern. That's the biggest difference. That's why we want to be very careful about our old patterns creeping up, as they are what's gotten us into the unhealthy habits we are fighting against today.

<u>Reasons or Excuses</u>

Now let's dig a little deeper. Those with a reason versus an excuse usually have a Plan B on how to get going again and/or how to get back on track. This is what I encourage my clients to do when they have "reasons" for missing the workout or the right eating habits. How do we learn from the prior situation? How do we pivot and how do we now move forward? If you are in the "excuse" zone, you will probably continue to direct the blame in other directions, away from yourself. This isn't healthy and will cause you to stay in that place for longer than you need to. Acknowledge, accept and move on.

It is dangerous to stay in that place because it is easy to fall into the victim mentality there. The victim mentality is what we mentioned above: you are the victim and everyone else is to blame. However, I believe and the Bible says you are the victor. There will be situations and circumstances that come against you, but you can overcome them all! "And they overcame him by the blood of the Lamb and by the word of their testimony, and they did not love their lives to the death." (Revelation 12:11).

One of the best ways to stay out of the "excuse zone," especially as it concerns your health and fitness is to set up systems and boundaries. Treat your health and wellness as seriously as you do other things like going to church—I hope you are going to church—your jobs or your children. Treat your health and fitness as non-negotiable. Do not to let things, situations, people or circumstances trample over your commitment and treat it without regard.

Let's think about it like this. I've heard this example taught, so I'm borrowing it for illustrative purposes. Say you have a safe deposit box with precious jewels, metals and even lots of cash. It belongs to you, however, you only have five of the six numbers to the combination lock to get in. Without the sixth number, you are not getting into the safe, even though the valuable items belong to you. Even though you have the other five numbers, you will not be able to redeem the valuable items until you get that sixth number.

Although other areas are flourishing in your life, until you make a commitment to your health and wellness, you will not experience the greatness inside of the safe deposit box that belongs to you. Your health and wellness are part of the heritage God designed and desires for you to have. You are the only one who can either prevent or allow that to happen.

Setting Boundaries

You are going to need to lay some groundwork with yourself and your loved ones as you go along this journey. It is always great to get the blessing of family and friends in this area, but understand if that doesn't happen, you still have to do what you have to do. You have to set boundaries and enforce them. Boundaries are needed from multiple sides. You need to set them so you don't cross areas that are not good or safe for you. You also have to set them so others don't cross into territory where you have not given them permission, or in their influence that won't be beneficial for you.

Understand, people are watching you, especially those closest to you. If they see that you let things continue to get in the way of your health and wellness, they will see that you are not taking this seriously and they won't take it seriously either. They will see and understand there is no boundary they must respect, because you haven't respected or enforced it. My belief is their lack of respect for your boundary usually isn't intentional. It is a natural response to your behavior.

When people see your discipline and mindset around this area being enforced by you, they too will respect your commitment in this area of your health and wellness. They won't have unreasonable expectations that you will ignore your health and wellness for them. In a similar way, they wouldn't think it reasonable for you to miss work for their less than urgent need.

Why? Because this is what brings in money and your actions have probably made that crystal clear that this is a boundary that you enforce, even without saying it.

I know that you are used to showing up for everyone. However, if your health is suffering from allowing it to be negotiable and meeting everyone else's needs, you won't be able to sustain it.

You won't be able to continue bringing in money from the business you can't say no to or it will slip out of your hands in other ways like costly insurance and prescription drugs. So, it is key to set the boundaries and enforce now to get ahead of the situation

I have distinct pictures in my head of two powerful women who tell stories about being protective over non-negotiable time. The first is an author who writes about having children who are constantly going non-stop. She has to continuously tend to their needs all day long, except for the set-apart time when everyone sees Mommy in the chair with the blanket over her head. They know that it is her non-negotiable time with Jesus, and interruptions are not acceptable. They know not to disturb her. She has trained them that whatever else is happening, other than the house burning down, don't interrupt her or there will be consequences. I love it! She has set a boundary and trained others, including and especially her children, to respect it. She doesn't break her rule, and she doesn't allow anyone else to interrupt or force their urgent need on her during this coveted time.

The second woman is a very successful speaker and money expert. I heard her share about a time when her assistant scheduled an important meeting with a famous media outlet during her recurring prayer meeting. She quickly corrected her assistant and didn't allow this seemingly important media outlet to meet with her at this "blocked-off" time. She did not allow her boundary around this coveted prayer time to be moved. I'm so glad this meeting with an esteemed media outlet didn't cause her to buckle under pressure for something that was a priority to her. I'm also glad that she didn't allow her assistant to dictate what was more important, or assume that it was okay to overstep this boundary. I'm sure her assistant learned an important lesson with this situation.

The take-away here is not only to enforce other's respecting your boundaries, but also to never skip an appointment with God. Because we are incorporating our faith into this journey, these are appointments with God too! What if we treated every workout as a meeting with God, as a time where we are not just moving our bodies, but we are moving heaven too. Because we are praying, worshiping, speaking to God, it's a non-negotiable appointment with God. How awesome is that?

Now I know that may sound a bit extreme, and maybe a little over-the-top, but why can't we be that way for the temples that God told us to glorify Him in? Who's willing to be that extreme and radical with your faith and fitness?

Let the Soaring Begin

This is part the where you walk out what you believe and talk like you believe it; where you really put action into place and live the kingdom lifestyle that you were created to live. This is where you begin to soar. Birds that soar can maintain flight without their wings flapping. They use the rising air currents. You have the ability to maintain this heightened and elevated lifestyle, without your wings flapping, without yoyo dieting, starting and stopping or not starting at all, by using your faith as your air currents. This is also where you are met with uncertain weather conditions, opposition, harsh terrain, etc. But this is also where you show the world what you are made of, your identity in Christ! Let's go!

Below are a few takeaways from Chapter One. You may choose to come back and reflect on these later.

Lessons:

A. The first step is always to acknowledge if there is a problem and make the decision to invite Christ in to help you solve it.

B. Know your "whys" and keep the vision before you at all times It is highly likely that you are going to want to quit. Don't be shocked when it happens, but be ready to respond. When it happens say, "Oh yeah! Coach April told me this would happen and now I know how to fight it."

C. Know you are worth a healthy lifestyle because you were bought with a heavy price. Take care of this expensive, luxury item called you! Stay committed, set boundaries, let go of any excuses.

Now we have identified a few lessons, let's couple them with scriptural confessions to apply these principles in your life in a practical way.

Repeat them several times or even take them as you would a medical prescription multiple times per day over a period of time until they become real in your heart.

We will have this exercise in each chapter because I believe the Word of God is alive and has a supernatural ability to change us if we allow it to. "For the word of God is living and powerful, and sharper than any two-edged sword." (Hebrews 4:12).

Embrace these scriptures and allow them to transform your life if you dare to believe them. Better yet make a decision to believe them! Notice the inclusion of "I/Me" because we need this to be personal and specific to YOU! Saying "I" brings you into the scripture.

<u>Confessions:</u>

- I am a new creation; old things have passed away; behold, I have become new. (2 Corinthians 5:17).

- Blessed be the God and Father of our Lord Jesus Christ, who has blessed me with every spiritual blessing in the heavenly places in Christ. (Ephesians 1:3).

- He chose me in Him before the foundation of the world, that I should be holy and without blame before Him in love. (Ephesians 1:4).

- In Him I have redemption through His blood, the forgiveness of sins, according to the riches of His grace. (Ephesians 1:7).

- Now, therefore, I am no longer a stranger and foreigner, but a fellow citizen with the saints and members of the household of God. (Ephesians 2:19).

Prayer:

Father,

Thank you for your unfailing love. You see my heart and know my thoughts. You see the decision I am making to choose a healthy kingdom lifestyle that glorifies you. I ask you accept my repentance for not stewarding my temple the way I should have and for your grace to help along this faith and fitness journey. Help me to set the proper realistic goals, to be committed this time for real, to you first, to me second, and to be a testimony to others around me. Give me the strength necessary to soar and the wisdom to make the right choices. I invite you onto the journey and I look forward to the great things that you have in store. I love you. In Jesus Name I Pray! Amen.

CHAPTER TWO

MINDSET MATTERS

<u>Keep Renewing Your Mind</u>

L et me be completely honest with you. This is an ongoing battle, probably daily, if not more often than that, but necessary to be successful in your faith and fitness goals. Because this is a lifestyle change decision, you will constantly have the enemy bombarding you with thoughts that just don't line up with what God has said about you. More on that when you get to the confession section. He's said some good stuff that I need you to hold on to.

In this stage, you must receive true freedom from every yoke of bondage—not just freedom from, but also freedom to. Believe your freedom comes with the new kingdom lifestyle changes you are making. You have freedom from the old ways of thinking and behaving in regards to your health and wellness, and freedom to live a more restricted, boundary filled, active life than you had before. You need to renew your mind from thinking you are missing out on something you used to have in the past and now can't have. This is what the enemy will try to get you to believe.

You have to see the foods that were bad for your health not as something you are missing out on. The sedentary life you lived on the couch in front of the TV is not something you are missing out on. You are free from it and freed to a healthier kingdom lifestyle. You are free to eat heathier and perhaps differently from others around you. So, be sure not to let others put you back in bondage because of your new choices. You need to be careful not to put yourself back in bondage in these areas as well.

You are free to have a new and vibrant lifestyle contrary to what's going on around you. If you continue with the mindset that you are missing out on something from the past that you haven't fully committed to let go of, you will always want it, because you will think you are missing out on something.

I encourage you not to live in the past constantly thinking about foods you used to love, which weren't fueling your body. There may be an opportunity for you to have that food again on special occasions. However, if banana pudding is your thing, look for ways, ideas, recipes, etc. to have it in a healthier manner that will fuel your body instead of tearing it down. Find a new way to make banana pudding, with less sugar and less processed ingredients. You can't live in the past. Remember, you are new creatures in Christ; the old has passed away. "Therefore, if anyone is in Christ, he is a new creation; old things have passed away; behold, all things have become new." (2 Corinthians 5:17). We really have to get a revelation of this in order to have lasting success on this faith and fitness journey; to really soar!

I have to fight through this as well. No-one who is serious about kingdom change in their lives is exempt from this if he or she is honest, really honest. The great thing as believers is we are given instructions on how to overcome. And this is the reason I have included the scripture confessions is because sometimes we just might forget. But that's okay because I have you covered!

At the Root of it All

Depending upon how you were raised or the various life experiences you have gone through, it may be more difficult to shift the way you filter and embrace things. However, renewing the mind is not just a nice to do; not "if I renew my mind" but "when I renew my mind." It's critical. The Bible is very clear that we must renew our minds, therefore it is non-negotiable. It's how you're going to stay focused; it's how you're going to see yourselves with the right identity; and it's how you're going to crush every lie of the enemy that says otherwise.

Not dealing with root issues can cause your body to operate under internalized stress, which could lead to emotional eating or depression, over compensation, self-preservation or even seeing yourselves in ways God didn't ordain, like ugly or fat or mean or whatever! All have harmful outcomes. In this case, you are not looking to God but believing the lie, so going back to the importance of mindset is crucial. If you don't get that right, it will be a continuous uphill battle. In my opinion this is the reason why so many Christians get off track. They start off fine, walking on the water. However, as soon as they take their eyes off Christ they begin to sink. Another failed diet, another workout DVD collecting dust; and another doctor's visit that ends with undesirable news.

Not everyone grew up in an amazing home with constant affirmations… I know I didn't. Not that my home was awful, however, there were definitely broken pieces that caused me to see myself in a light that wasn't always bright and shining. Lack of confidence issues took root at an early age, which I have to body slam constantly, over and over and over again. (I was a wrestling-watcher with my brothers growing up).

There are words that affect us, especially at a young age. The old saying "sticks and stones may break your bones but words will never hurt," is a lie from the pit of hell. There are words, curses spoken every day, whether we choose to believe it or not. If we don't deal with them and address them, they can affect us in ways we may not realize. Comfort eating, stress eating, binge eating, no eating, all stem from an unhealthy self-image. Often-times they are a result of what we heard someone say, which wasn't God's truth about us. God says you are fearfully and wonderfully made. "I will praise You, for I am fearfully and wonderfully made; Marvelous are Your works, And that my soul knows very well." (Psalm 139:14). Praise Him! Make sure your soul knows that! Don't look around at others, don't look to the TV, magazine or social media to validate this truth. God said it, believe it. Meditate, meaning think about and ponder this scripture daily on your faith and fitness journey and see how things change. You will be amazed!

At the ripe age of ten, I experienced my first battle with body shaming that caused me to struggle with feeling fat throughout my teens and some of my adult life. A boy called me "big." This wasn't just any boy. This was someone I thought was super cute and had a little crush on at the time. His words shattered me and rang over and over and over in my ears for years. I would constantly replay "he said I was big" and if he said it, it must be true, because that is what he saw. This hindered me from wearing certain clothes and participating in certain activities I thought I was "too big" to engage in. However, what looks permanent can have a sudden turnaround in Him.

The Foundation

Laying the proper foundation is critical. If this journey is not built on Christ, it won't stand, as the scriptures tell us. The winds will blow and the only house that stands will be the one built on the solid rock. "Therefore whoever hears these sayings of Mine, and does them, I will liken him to a wise man who built his house on the rock: and the rain descended, the floods came, and the winds blew and beat on that house; and it did not fall, for it was founded on the rock. But everyone who hears these sayings of Mine, and does not do them, will be like a foolish man who built his house on the sand: and the rain descended, the floods came, and the winds blew and beat on that house; and it fell. And great was its fall." (Matthew 7:24-27).

Sure, others do it without Christ, but their foundation is not solid and the house won't stand even if it looks good from every angle on the outside. Even if it doesn't manifest in their health, wellness or fitness, it is guaranteed to manifest in another way. Their relationships, their jobs, their whatever! So, my plea to you is to be wise and not foolish. Listen to the words of Jesus and not only hear them but do them. Build your faith and fitness journey on His solid foundation.

The thing about foundations is they are not super cool or cute to look at and therefore it is easy for the average person to skip over them. I mean, come on, think about it, when was the last time you walked past a new home or building being built and said or even thought to yourself, "Oh my goodness, look at that foundation, it's amazing!" or "that foundation is so cool, it's flat and sturdy." Let's be honest, you probably haven't, but when the home or building is complete, the admiration is magnified. You may talk about the brick or the siding or the windows or even the landscape around it. None of these has anything to do with the building standing and doing what it was designed to do, but the foundation does!

Neither the beauty of the structure nor the underwhelming appearance of the foundation changes the importance of the foundation being solid and necessary. If the home or building fell, who would remember how beautiful it was? All you would probably think about is "What kind of builder put down a faulty foundation?" or "Oh my goodness, who doesn't know that the foundation has to be strong before you build on it?" Everyone knows that the foundation is the most important part of a structure.

Now, think about your journey. Can you now envision the need for a proper foundation? You don't just want to be pretty, or just skinny, or just anything. You want the proper foundation so that other things won't fall and crumble. I tell my clients all the time, you don't just want to lose weight, you want to transform!

I'm sure you have heard it said that if one were to look at your schedule and credit/bankcard/receipts, it would be obvious where your heart was. It would show which things are important to you. The Bible is clear about where your heart and your treasure are. The things you are willing to invest in show where your priorities lie and what's important to you. "For where your treasure is, there your heart will be also." (Matthew 6:21). I'm always so saddened by people who say they can't afford to make their health a priority.

If you are not putting time or money behind your health and wellness now, you will definitely do so in the future - many times over, through doctor visits and prescription medication when things are not working the way that they should. It's like maintaining a car. You have to put in money for regular maintenance, oil changes, tire rotations and the like. Maintaining these items prevents larger, higher priced problems from occurring.

When people tell me that gym memberships are too expensive, a trainer is too expensive, they can't afford it, or worst of all, it's too expensive to eat healthy food, I want to take out their bank statement or credit card and show them where they are putting their value. I actually will do this in my programs to show people they actually do have the time and the money. They just need the proper mindset or foundation and commitment. It does take an investment. If you legitimately don't have the money, start with walking - it's free. Buy less processed foods and drink more water. There are countless things you can do for free to debunk the "expensive: myth.

You're Not Your Past

Old baggage will weigh you down. I know some of us may have grown up with traumatic experiences and these must be dealt with on a higher level. There is nothing wrong with that. Please don't feel ashamed to get the help you need. I totally believe in inner healing. Part of that inner healing comes with solidifying your identity in Christ and not your identity from your past. This doesn't mean that you have to hide from your past. There is probably a story in you because of your past, but you cannot allow your past to keep you in the past.

If you are not healed from your past, you run the risk of falling into the victim mentality. This not a good place to be. If undealt with, it can crush you and cause the cycle all over again and this is not a life that you or anyone one really wants to live. I know because I have been there before. And I'm guessing this is a battle you may have faced before too. Now it's time to say, "No more!" You can't let this muscle get any stronger. You are focusing on a new muscle today! Both in your natural bodies and your spirit!

No more holding yourself hostage to your past! Jesus said, "It is finished!" on the cross at Calvary! He has already paid the price for you! "So when Jesus had received the sour wine, He said, 'It is finished!' And bowing His head, He gave up His spirit." (John 19:30). Don't make His work of no effect by looking anywhere other than the cross. God sees you crowned with glory and honor. "You have made him a little lower than the angels; You have crowned him with glory and honor, And set him over the works of Your hands." (Hebrews 2:7)

Whew, now that is powerful! Read that again. You've seen someone else, another vision, that's double vision or two visions which also equals division. Don't be divided from Christ. Get His vision, then take captive every thought to the obedience of Christ, keeping your mindset right. "Casting down arguments and every high thing that exalts itself against the knowledge of God, bringing every thought into captivity to the obedience of Christ." (2 Corinthians 10:5).

You also can't allow your past to keep you on a hamster wheel of self-destructive, self-sabotaging behavior. For years, I didn't share the insecurity of believing I was fat because a boy whom I liked when I was ten years old called me big. Do you hear me? I was ten! This plagued me for years. It prevented me from soaring for years. I allowed this lie to weigh me down until I received the truth of what and who God said I am. Finally, I changed the narrative and my faulty belief system. I no longer have to hide behind the lie "I'm too big!" Instead, today I hide behind the scripture "I'm fearfully and wonderfully made," as mentioned earlier in Psalm 139!

Situations like this, or worse, may cause you to withdraw when you are speaking, or to overeat when you are feeling super-emotional or stressed out. You may try use your situation to get back at the person who hurt you. I know it sounds strange, but sometimes we do things to ourselves with the misconception that it will hurt someone who hurt us, only to find we actually only afflicted ourselves. Now, I'm not a psychologist, but I have done and seen these behaviors in myself and my clients, so I'm familiar enough.

This leads me to the next point. As I stated earlier, you want true transformation, transformation that starts on the inside and works outward. The Bible says we are transformed by renewing our minds. "And do not be conformed to this world, but be transformed by the renewing of your mind, that you may prove what *is* that good and acceptable and perfect will of God." (Romans 12:2). Sure, you want to lose weight, however if that transformation on the inside never takes place, the weight will rear its ugly head again. It really takes leaning on your faith not to go down this road again. When you do transform, you are in God's perfect will for your life! Isn't that amazing? Definitely something to be excited about!

This means that you can't lost weight just to please someone else who thinks you should without the right intent, that's a wrong motive. That is different from doing it for your "whys." When you are doing it for your "whys," you are doing it for those you are called to support and live a long life to impact them. You are also doing this to walk in God's will for your life and not wanting to lose weight because of a manipulative spirit that doesn't have your best interest at heart, but only wants to shame you or make you feel bad.

You can't soar in your faith and fitness for that type of person. If you do, you will always revert, because your "why" isn't strong enough; it's to please rather than impact. If the person or people aren't building you up and encouraging you in the right way, you need to separate from them no matter what the relationship is. If the person's behavior causes you to be depressed or stressed, that is a sure sign of a boundary that is lacking or has been overstepped. Create or reinforce one fast, and keep your distance for your own healthy success!

When my clients tell me things like "I was able to pray away my fear and doubt and go from zero sit ups to fourteen" or "I feel like I want to keep going" through my programs, those are key indicators that change and growth are taking place. The past is no longer gripping them, but their faith is beginning to mold them! This not only makes me the proudest coach, but it also helps me help them use this as more fuel in the gas tank to keep going. Use this to stir up and create the passion for change that is inside of every one of us. It just needs to be ignited. Or, if you had it once before, get your passion back. Be in faith, be a dreamer with God!

Overwhelm

Don't allow this process to overwhelm you and again take you out. For sure, emotions will fly. There will be mountain tops and valley lows. However, stick with it and conquer your emotions. If you begin to feel overwhelmed, dial it back a little. Start off with smaller, attainable goals and build from there.

Overwhelm tends to kick in when you try to do too much and in your own strength. This is why you are encouraged to lean on your faith in this health and fitness lifestyle change. It's why this process is different from anything else you may have tried in the past. It is not just about willpower. Your will certainly is involved, but it's also knowing and understanding you can go to your Heavenly Father when you are feeling overwhelmed, even with your health, wellness and fitness goals.

We all know in our heads that we are to trust in the Lord and not our own understanding. This is a familiar scripture, but how often do we really do it? And the last part is usually left off completely, but no more, the time is now. "Trust in the Lord with all your heart, and lean not on your own understanding; in all your ways acknowledge Him, And He shall direct your paths. Do not be wise in your own eyes; Fear the Lord and depart from evil." (Proverbs 3:5-7).

He is near and He is listening as well as ready to step in on your behalf. Jesus urges us to come to Him with our problems, our burdens, and He will help. We can rest in Him: "Come to Me, all you who labor and are heavy laden, and I will give you rest." (Matthew 11:28). Allow Him to help you!

God promises to help you. He promises to be there for you. "God is our refuge and strength, A very present help in trouble." (Psalm 46:1) Trust that and go to Him every time you are in need on this journey. I don't believe He will put more on you than you can handle. He will even make a way of escape for you to be able to bear any temptation. "No temptation has overtaken you except such as is common to man; but God is faithful, who will not allow you to be tempted beyond what you are able, but with the temptation will also make the way of escape, that you may be able to bear it." (1 Corinthians 10:13). God is for you, He is on your side, and He is pulling for you to crush this thing once and for all. You just have to be willing to bring Him along on the journey.

You Are Worth Fighting For

Have you ever heard that song *Worth Fighting For* by Brian Courtney Wilson? (God speaks to me a lot through song so you will hear several examples as you read along). If not, I recommend you go put this book down now—I give you permission. Go and listen to it. It's not a recent song, but as my Pastor would say, "It's an oldie but goodie!" It basically breaks down how God believes we are worth fighting for. There is a part in the song that quotes the scripture about eye hasn't not seen, ear hasn't heard all that the Lord has planned for those who love Him. "Eye has not seen, nor ear heard, Nor have entered into the heart of man the things which God has prepared for those who love Him." (1 Corinthians 2:9).

There is so much still worth fighting for - your health, the kingdom, your peace - they are all worth fighting for. Then the song declares that victory is mine. Whew, so good, so good, so good! So, I speak that song over you right now and I pray that whenever times get hard you will stop what you are doing and find a way to listen to that song, and get to renewing your mind again. It encourages me every time and I have a dance party!

Believing this really and truly will be key to your success on this journey and all of life.

God already picked you, hand-picked you and called you His very own. He did it because He believed you were worth fighting for! I remember the day I sat in Coach White's Office. He had a reputation for being tough and sometimes a hot-head. But it didn't matter to me. I thought he was cute and his girls' varsity basketball team was fire! I heard the announcement in A period that he was looking for a manager for the team. I thought to myself, "I want to do this! I'm going to go talk to Coach White and let him know I'm interested."

Soon after, I ran into him in passing on my way to class and mentioned that I wanted to speak with him about something. He agreed and told me when to come to his office. The time came and I was kind-of excited as I sat there with a big smile on my face, sitting across from this super cute man whom I would have the pleasure of seeing more frequently once I became manager of the team (This was BC and I was young y'all before you judge me haha). I'm sure the suspense was only built up in my mind! I was ready to burst out with excitement and share with him why I had wanted to meet with him. My confidence was high; I knew I would be great for the job, so my mouth opened and I told him I wanted to be the manager for the girls' varsity basketball team. I wasn't quite ready for his response though.

"Why do you want to be the manager? Why don't you play instead?" was his response. Hmm, what? He wasn't quite following the plan I had set out in my mind. "Just show up to free play on Monday morning at 6:30 am and we can go from there." "Ummmm, excuse me," I thought in my head... I was speechless. I didn't know how to respond. I wasn't a basketball player. I was more of the cheerleader type, at least I thought I was. This was not what I had expected; this was not a part of the plan!

However, the conversation was pretty much over and guess who was at Free Play at 6:30 am on Monday morning (sigh)! I didn't feel bamboozled though. I actually felt kind of proud. He saw something in me and put a smile on my face that day. That was freshman year and I guess the beginning of my journey as an athlete... well not really. I landed on the Freshman B Team! But when I heard that I had ninth period practice instead of gym I was sold! I'm going to make some people smile right now — that meant no more mandatory swimming in gym class and terrible hair days. Glory!

The moral of this story is it's great when someone sees something in you and picks you, but it's so much greater when God picks you, and beloved, He already has, even before the foundation of the world. "Just as He chose us in Him before the foundation of the world, that we should be holy and without blame before Him in love." (Ephesians 1:4). And now He is giving you the opportunity to pick you too!

I totally get it when scriptures talk about man looking at the outward appearance but God judging the heart. However, I think we hide behind that scripture to justify when we know our outward appearance may not be quite where it should be. (I'm sure to get some nasty letters and emails behind this one, but please, please, please, okay one more please, hear my heart).

Now, don't get me wrong, your outside should never be more put-together than your inside, because God is judging the heart. And Paul was clear that exercise was important, but not that important. (LOL) "For bodily exercise profits a little, but godliness is profitable for all things, having promise of the life that now is and of that which is to come." (1 Timothy 4:8). Paul wasn't saying don't exercise or only a little, but not to make it more important than godliness. My appeal to you is that both your inside - when you pursue godliness - and your outside – when you pursue health can look good and be pleasing to God first, and pleasing to you! This is part of self-care, which we will discuss later. It's also part of knowing and celebrating your value and worth!

Part of the process of renewing your mind is believing this truth. You are worth fighting for. Jesus proved that on the cross. He did His part. He gave up His life for you. Who else would and could do that for you? "Greater love has no one than this, than to lay down one's life for his friends." (John 15:13). Or better yet, can you visualize Him fighting for you and on your behalf? Think about the attacks of the enemy coming at you, all the fiery darts coming at you, and the Lord shields you behind Himself and He wards off all the attacks of the enemy—like you would protect a child in the midst of harm and danger if he or she called out for your help. Think about that—He is shielding you!

Now, the flip side of that is you doing your part. You also have to fight for you! Believe that YOU are worth fighting for and fight. Fight for your health and wellness, to own it, to take it back! Now I am definitely not one who subscribes to the unscriptural claim that God helps those who help themselves. However, I am a firm believer of the Word that faith without works is dead! "For as the body without the spirit is dead, so faith without works is dead also." (James 2:26). I believe you have to walk by faith—that's when you don't see it. But the walking part to me is the works part. You don't just stand still in faith.

You are in a battle for your health and wellness. Again, salvation goes beyond just going to heaven. And if the enemy comes only to steal, kill and destroy, what do you think he is doing if he didn't get you at the salvation piece? But praise God, the next part talks about the role Christ played. He came that you would have life and have it more abundantly. (John 10:10). If you are stricken with illness and inflammation and stuck on medication or find it hard to move, or have no energy, is that really abundant life? You have to fight for you!

In the getting started phase, we discussed you having to be your number one fan, your biggest cheerleader, your own superhero, even if no-one here on this earth decides to join you. Well, this is necessary in the renewing your mind phase too because you are constantly fighting. Let go of any past baggage; get over it when your husband, momma or bestie won't do it with you, or worse, won't support you in your endeavors.

It will suck when the people closest to you are not supportive or not fighting for you as much as you would like. However, remember this is Lord's battle. He will fight for you if you are in position. You have to do your part, the part that the Lord is clearly speaking to you about in this hour. It takes time to know what He is saying and then obeying. "If you are willing and obedient, you shall eat the good of the land." (Isaiah 1:19). If no one ever supports you, you have to believe beyond a shadow of a doubt that you are worth fighting for. Your health and wellness are worth fighting for. Then be willing to obey what He is leading you to do to be healthy and well.

See yourself with the power of the Holy Spirit in you and nothing can stop you. It's going to take a clear mindset shift. And I have every belief that you can and will do it! Faith and prayer are going to be your fitness superpower support.

Once you make this decision, you are in a good place. This will become one of your "whys" and obviously you are another "why." Keep fighting for you! The good news is that it's not impossible or unattainable. You are on the right path and the more you keep pushing, the more progress you will make. The more progress you make better you will feel. Accomplishment feels wonderful!

Below are a few takeaways from Chapter Two. You may choose to come back and reflect on these later.

Lessons:

A. Don't let your past dictate your future. Keep fighting to renew your mind each and every day. Get to the root of the thing and kill it. Ask God for inner healing in these deep-rooted areas.

B. Set the proper foundation and believe in your worth! God thought you worthy enough to send His Son to die for you, now you must believe you are worthy enough to make the health decisions necessary to soar.

C. You are worth fighting for. Don't allow this process to overwhelm you and stop you in your tracks.

Confessions:

- I cast down arguments and every high thing that exalts itself against the knowledge of God, I bring every thought into captivity to the obedience of Christ. (2 Corinthians 10:5).

- I am renewed in the Spirit of my mind. (Ephesians 4:23).

- I present my body as a living sacrifice, holy, acceptable to God, which is my reasonable service. (Romans 12:1).

- I am not conformed to this world, but I am transformed by the renewing of my mind, that I may prove what is that good and acceptable and perfect will of God. (Romans 12:2).

Prayer:

Father,

I ask You to help me to renew my mind; to see things differently from how I have in the past; to see myself as you see me; to see my body how you see it; to see food as a source of nourishment to fuel my body and not as a comfort or escape mechanism. Show me how to trust you and leave the past behind, because it does not define me. I choose to press forward toward the prize and deal with any unresolved issues so they don't manifest again. Thank you for hand-picking me and revealing more of the greatness you have placed inside me. When I feel overwhelmed, I will run to you instead of things that won't do me good. Help me remember that you believe I am worth fighting for, so I will do the same and continue fighting too! In Jesus Name I Pray! Amen.

CHAPTER THREE

YOU ARE WORTH IT

Don't Go for the Lie

S ometimes the thing that keeps knocking us down is feeling unworthy but as we just discussed, you are worth fighting for. And if God sent His only begotten Son to die for you then you certainly are worthy. "For God so loved the world that He gave His only begotten Son, that whoever believes in Him should not perish but have everlasting life." (John 3:16). When people don't feel worthy, they are actually thinking and believing God doesn't think they are worthy or doesn't love them. That couldn't be further from the truth. After all, He bought us with a price!

When you don't believe you are worthy, you don't understand what Jesus did at the cross and that brings us back to decision-making back in Chapter One and renewing the mind in Chapter Two. You can't ask Him to go back to the cross. If you have been saved for any amount of time, you will know that it was finished at the cross.

What are you saying to yourself? What thoughts are you letting rule you? There is always a lie the enemy will use to prevent you from starting, or to keep you off track. However, you can choose not to partner with that lie.

The book of Jeremiah declares that God is thinking good thoughts about you. If you weren't worthy or worth it, then He wouldn't be thinking good thoughts about you. He wouldn't have predestined a plan for your life. No matter what you have experienced up until this point, it won't change the truth of His Word. "'For I know the thoughts that I think toward you,' says the Lord, 'thoughts of peace and not of evil, to give you a future and a hope. Then you will call upon Me and go and pray to Me, and I will listen to you. And you will seek Me and find Me, when you search for Me with all your heart.'" (Jeremiah 29:11-13).

And guess what? I have another song that helps me when I have listened to the lie. I believe it will help you too. It's called *Come Away With Me* by Jesus Culture. The song title alone supports the notion in this book's subtitle: Invite God in on the Journey.

However, when you listen to the lyrics, it goes on to say that God has a plan for you that is going wild, it's going to be great and full of Him! Whew, isn't that exciting? No way would you call someone to come away with you if that person wasn't very valuable to you. He says to call upon Him and pray to Him and He will listen! God wants to give you a future and a hope! It's not too late! Be encouraged, Beloved, be encouraged!

<u>Belief in You</u>

Earlier I gave the example of Coach White seeing something in me that he thought I should play basketball versus be the team manager. Again, nothing wrong with being the manager. Every team needs a manager. But I wonder if what he saw in me was a fear of stepping out. Perhaps he saw something in me that I just didn't see in myself, something I didn't believe until his nudge confronted my fear.

Okay, I have another basketball example. Joe was one of the students I met many years ago in our college campus outreach ministry. Although Joe didn't play on the school's basketball team, he loved to play basketball and would participate in pickup games when he could, amidst his busy engineering class schedule. When Joe found out I used to play basketball in high school, his face lit. There was something that turned up in him and from that day forward Joe encouraged me to get back into the game.

Joe would often say things like "I bet if you trained now, you could try out for the WNBA." Ha, now I was a scrub in high school, remember Freshman B team, and I didn't play my senior year or in college! However, beyond flattery, Joe encouraged me so much and in such a way that in the back of my mind I really wondered if he could be right. There was a tiny glimpse of hope that, if I put in the work, if I put in the work, okay let me say that one more time for the people in the back, if I put in the work and discipline, it could pay off.

Whether or not I pick up a ball again, Joe's voice in the back of my head resonates with an internal confidence that "maybe I can." To this day, if I even see a basketball, I smile and think about Joe. I think about his desire to inspire and see greatness in me. I want to do the same for others.

Now, I didn't feel like the WNBA was something God was telling me to do, pursue or believe Him for, but my point here is oftentimes someone will see a worth in you that you can agree with and begin to see in yourself. This is sometimes the push you need to see your value. This is the self-worth I try to instill in each of my clients. I see value in them. More importantly, God sees value in them and you too!

Self-care

Knowing who you are in Christ is self-care. When you really, truly start to believe God's Word and what He says about you and your worth, your actions will align with it. When we see the value of something, we go all out for it and treat it with the utmost care. Consider one the parables Jesus shared about the kingdom. The merchant that found the one pearl of great price sold all that he had just to buy it. He deemed the great value and went all in to get it. "Again, the kingdom of heaven is like a merchant seeking beautiful pearls, who, when he had found one

pearl of great price, went and sold all that he had and bought it."
(Matthew 13:45-46) You are that pearl worth a great price. Don't
be afraid to see, share and invest in your value.

Recently I have been all about quotes. And one of my new
favorites is "Eating healthy is a sign of respect." Because you
have the utmost respect for your body, you treat it with the
utmost care and feed it with things that are not only going to
help it, but won't harm it either. This journey will definitely
involve making better decisions. It's like saying something runs
like a "well-oiled machine." It runs well because it is "well-
oiled," meaning it is taken care of and it functions at an optimal
level because of the care put into it. Our bodies are the same.
When we take care of them, they perform at an optimal level;
when we don't, they don't. It's simple!

You don't put anything else other than gas in your car because
you KNOW it's the only thing that will make the car run. If you
put other things in it, like water, or worse, sugar, do you think it
will run? Absolutely not! Sugar will not allow your car to run
and it won't cause your body to function at its highest potential
either. There is much to be said about sugar and how harmful it
is for your body, your immune system and so much more.
However, I will have to save that for another book. (Sigh)

Another good quote is "Your health is your wealth," which I
mentioned earlier. If you are healthy, you can go places; if you
aren't, you won't. If you have joint problems and back problems,

inflammation and sickness in your body, that isn't wealth. You are unable to do the great things you were destined to do, because these things are hindering you. That is not wealth; that is detriment.

Know Who and Whose You Are

Again, once you know who you are, you will begin to behave and act like the royalty you are designed to be. You won't fall back into the ordinary life that caused you to eat things that don't fuel your body, or to live a sedentary life. You do this by building your identity in Christ! Once the prodigal son realized who His father was, which in turn affected who he was and what he had access to, he went home! It's time to go home, and that is why we invite God in on this journey.

Important to note here because we have to keep that mindset right as discussed in the previous chapter, the prodigal son did NOT say, "What if this doesn't work?" "What if my father doesn't let me come back?" He knew who his father was; he knew what his father had; and he knew his father's authority. You too must have the same revelation on this journey, of who your father is, thus who you are!

Knowing who your Father is, is knowing that He is here to help you. Knowing what your Father has means knowing He has the resources for you to be successful on your fitness journey. Knowing your Father's authority means knowing that, when the enemy comes in to try and tempt you with the old ways and behaviors, or tell you the lie that this time won't work either, you have tried this in the past and failed, you can kick him out, because your Father has given you authority as His child.

You need to realize we are in a race and we are running for the prize. Without action, your words alone won't get you there. God has been talking to me a lot about faith without works being dead. So, let's keep running, let's keep changing, let's obtain the prize God has for us in our health and wellness.

I believe everyone should be able to look in the mirror and smile because they are pleased with the person God created. Doesn't mean that we don't have flaws, doesn't mean we are perfect, but means we are confident in who God created us to be! Self-care covers a lot of different areas, not just the spa, or shopping, or dinner with your friends. Self-care does include relieving and avoiding stress and creating boundaries. Most importantly, it doesn't exist when the act is no longer beneficial to your health and wellness.

Self-care is not living a life lacking greatness. A sedentary life, high blood pressure, diabetes, high cholesterol or thirty different medications to stay in an unhealthy place is not self-care—and this isn't about man judging the outward appearance. That's a cop out! It is not taking personal responsibility for decisions we have made to get us here.

Heart disease and stroke are the number one killers among Americans; and disproportionally affects many ethnic groups to according to the American Heart Association (www.heart.org). But we can change this! As mentioned earlier, God clearly tells us to glorify Him in our bodies and I don't think the afore-mentioned ailments glorify Him!

For those of you who are thinking—because I can hear your thoughts—"some of these things are hereditary" or "my cousin who is seven was born with diabetes," to you I say, "it's time to break the curse, because Jesus paid the price." If you didn't have anything to do with it and it was simply passed down to you, send it back to hell. That's not your address. Pray and stand and use your faith for complete healing.

My point here is we still have to do our part and take action on the things we are able to control. Some of us have been hiding behind the hereditary door for too long, as well hoping we don't get found out. I say today "No more." Confess the scriptures outlined in these pages and command the enemy to flee! "Submit to God. Resist the devil and he will flee from you." (James 4:7)

Inside and Out

For those of you who take this to the other extreme, it is not healthy or God's perfect plan for you to be over-obsessed with your outward appearance. The Bible says you are fearfully and wonderfully made (which I have mentioned several times already so that it sinks in), you are the apple of His eye, His Beloved. So, I do think there is a healthy pleasure in believing what God says about you, but the enemy loves to take things to the extreme and have us out of balance. If you are on either end of the spectrum, reel it back in. If your doctor has given you a clean bill of health, and you are listening to your body, share this information with someone else to impact others.

For my super religious folks out there, I'm in no way suggesting that your physical health comes before your spiritual health. I think you can have both. So, keep glorifying God in your bodies and honor the fact that you have been bought with a price and your body is not your own. That means you can't do whatever you like to it and think it's okay. I know I keep mentioning this, but it's because I believe it is so important for us to understand. Repetition puts things into long term memory and this is a foundational principle upon which I have built my health and wellness business.

What if you truly surrendered in this area? What if you took the position that God's will is more precious than having your own way? I believe God would honor a heart and prayer like that, one that is not about you, but all about Him!

Below are a few takeaways from Chapter Three. You may choose to come back and reflect on these later.

Lessons:

A. It means the world when someone sees something in us that we may not see in ourselves. Use this as motivation and allow God to speak your worth to you through it.

B. It's okay to be pushed out of your comfort zone. Becoming comfortable with being uncomfortable stretches you, grows you and teaches you so much, inwardly and outwardly.

C. Take care of yourself. Your health is your wealth. Your plans can shift at any moment if you are open and ready for it; don't let it take you by surprise.

<u>Confessions:</u>

- I am His workmanship, created in Christ Jesus for good works, which God prepared beforehand that I should walk in them. (Ephesians 2:10).

- He chose me in Him before the foundation of the world, that I should be holy and without blame before Him in love. (Ephesians 1:4).

- Now, therefore, I am no longer a stranger and foreigner, but a fellow citizen with the saints and members of the household of God. (Ephesians 2:19).

- I am washed, I am sanctified, I am justified in the name of the Lord Jesus and by the Spirit of our God. (1 Corinthians 6:11).

<u>Prayer:</u>

Father,

I am so grateful that I belong to you. It amazes me that you loved me enough to send your Son to redeem me. It makes me feel wonderful when others see qualities and worth in me, but I ask you to help me see those things in myself. Heal me from the inside out and show me how to incorporate a proper balance of self-care. I know that it is not all about me and there is a bigger picture you are painting. I trust the work of your hands and the outcome of your masterpiece. You are the potter and I am the clay! I belong to you and choose not to believe the lies of the enemy. I will cast them down every time they surface and choose to believe what your Word says about me instead, meditating on it day and night as the scriptures instruct me. Thank you for these confessions that I have on hand and the many more promises outlined in the Bible. I will use them to fight and win! In Jesus Name I Pray! Amen

CHAPTER FOUR

RESILIENCE

When I Don't Feel Like It

D o you know how many times I and others who incorporate any kind of regular fitness routine into their lives has "felt like it"? Most of the time people don't work out because they feel like it; rather they do it because they have to, need to, must, it's necessary. It's part of the life they have chosen and they want the results. It's more important than the unhealthy alternative, and so on and so on. Many, like myself, have been on both sides of the fence - and like this side better. Plus, what do your feelings have to do with anything? They aren't the boss of you! LOL

I remember the day God gave me the Three P's when I didn't want to work out. "Be prepared, be positive, be protective." I thought this was so corny, but then it began to resonate with me in a great way. You have to be prepared! I recommend my clients prepare a workout bag before leaving the house; schedule your workouts; get your meals prepped for the week—all examples of being prepared! Personally, I had to incorporate the "no sit down" rule when I came home from work and still needed to go to the gym. I knew if I sat down even for a second it was over.

I used to have a coach who would say, "Embrace the suck!" Now I say the "suc" is necessary for to the "cess" in your success. If you go into this journey knowing not every day will be easy breezy, that will help when the sucky days come, because they will come. You can just acknowledge it: "Okay, this is when Coach April told me I wouldn't want to do it. Got it!" And then move on! This includes embracing and trusting the help of the accountability system you put in place, i.e. your coach, the Holy Spirit, others who have gone before you, etc. There is wisdom in that. You have to trust them and the process, even if it doesn't look quite like what you expected. Even when you don't quite understand why you feel the way you do, or why something is being asked of you, don't quite understand how it's related, please trust the process!

Again, being completely honest with you, not a ton of people really like to work out. Some do, but I would venture to say without any research that the majority don't. We like the results of working out and that is what I want to instill. I mean, you feel good and accomplished afterwards, but actually going through it, ugh! I include myself here too. I guarantee the emotions will fly! One day you will be like the little engine who could and another day you will be like the kid running because the school bully is after you and you just don't feel like fighting today. We need the results—and that's when we tell our mind and our body to shut up because we *are* going in this direction. No longer will you allow your mind to be in control.

Think about athletes, even Olympians, when they train. They have become so disciplined because they have their eyes on the prize, not the chocolate cake! Temptations cannot take their eyes off the prize. That is the type of faith, determination and grit that you have to have. You can't continue to look back and think about how good peach cobbler is. You have think about the long-term destruction that banana pudding is having on your health!

Market Research

Not too long ago I did some market research. I really wanted to serve my clients better and know how to speak to other kingdom women whom I had not yet reached. In a private or semi-private group, I asked the women who were believers why they didn't exercise and eat healthy even though they knew they should. I was going out on a limb, but I was curious as to how people would respond. Actually, I wasn't sure if anyone would respond. Oh boy, to my surprise there were almost two hundred and fifty comments back and forth on this topic.

I heard everything under the sun. Things like:

"I don't have support with the kids."

"Don't have the time or energy."

"I'm single and I don't like to cook."

"I'm lazy."

"I'm tired."

"I haven't put a priority on it."

"I live with people and have to eat what they eat."

"I don't have the money."

"I don't have the community."

"I don't have the time."

"We have mold in the house." HUH?

And so on and so on and so on. I was so grateful that so many people responded. I was overjoyed that they were totally open and honest with me. There was a lot of good information there that I could really use. But the other part of me was super sad. My heart was heavy. I was hurting for those women who were not soaring, not living their best kingdom life, and for the most part seemed okay with that. They knew they should care and do something about it, but they didn't. They didn't have a strong "why".

Once again I saw so many people, especially women, knowing they "should" and not doing it. Some were hiding behind fear; some were hiding behind money or lack thereof when it's free to walk and run all day long; some were hiding behind not knowing where to start, or lack of community. Each of them indicated they were believers in Jesus, which means they have access to Him; and the Holy Spirit, their teacher, lives inside them. However, it didn't appear that they were using this accessible weapon to own and control their health and wellness.

What I heard appeared to be a ton of excuses instead of legitimate reasons. I mean, I did hear a few reasons related to health and of course I recommended they work with their doctors to decide the best plan of action. But to do nothing when you know you should seems negligent to me. I believe we will stand before God and give an account of what we have done, as the Bible states. I think our health and wellness will be on the list of things we either stewarded well or handled without regard, and that is not okay. God has a better plan for you than that.

One woman openly admitted she didn't realize she was that far gone—and that's okay. Realizing it and not doing anything about it is the dangerous piece. Going about everyday activities and not acknowledging even the smallest fire is burning in the house is detrimental!

I went on to ask a follow up question but didn't get much response. It was a valid question about scripture instructing us we should take care of our bodies, the temples of the Holy Spirit. Can you imagine how that hurts the Father? In addition, the world should be envious of us, about how amazing our health is. We need to live in the "No excuse" zone.

Forward Motion

One of my biggest pet peeves is when people say they will "try," which gives a way out of putting in any real effort. It's a way to appease someone or be dishonest with themselves by saying, "I may put in some effort but if it doesn't work, I may just stop and say it didn't work." At least I can say I tried and it didn't work. I instill into my clients to incorporate saying "I will work at it" instead of "I'm trying." This actually forces you to put some skin in the game and really "work" towards the goal at hand. Trying requires minimum effort; working towards the goal requires continuous effort!

Taking baby steps is okay. Babies wobble when starting out. They fall down, get back up and go at it again. Babies don't stay on the floor crawling forever, even if the crawling period lasts longer than desired. Baby steps are steps forward, closer to the goal. You will continue to grow and get there eventually if you keep at it. Doing nothing is defeat.

Now, don't get me wrong. You will have days where you are going to be tired of the meal prepping or eating another piece of fish, and it will be easier to go to the fast-food joint. Push past the feelings and keep at it to "taste and see" the results. You won't like every recipe you try. You will have days where you are sore and don't want to work out again. You will have days where you are just hungry and don't want to eat right, but keep at it. If you to get off track, reset quickly. Get back on track immediately!

At this time, you may need to go back to your "whys." You will also have to push yourself. Push past the feelings, take rulership over your body. I once saw a quote that said, "Don't let your mind bully your body." I love that so much because it goes back to the purpose of renewing your mind. This feeling doesn't have to be your reality. Your actions are reality. Who is really in control? Don't allow your mind to tell your body it's okay for you to sit on the couch eating chips and sugary drinks. Your body has to rise up and say no more --- mind, we are getting out and walking today, we are going to this HIIT class, we are eating these vegetables and so on. Debo was so effective because he was bigger and stronger, just like your body!

So, suit up and let's go! Let's get on that treadmill that may have collected dust in the basement, that elliptical, or simply on the floor and do some good old-fashioned sit ups. Let's get an accountability partner and a system you will embrace and stick to. This will be key during these times. Let's go!

Fight For It

Know that you were built for this. If not, God wouldn't have told you to glorify Him in your body. He wouldn't ask you to do something you weren't capable of doing. Sometimes it boils down to how bad you want it. Other times it's about not being punked out of your destiny.

For many years, I didn't see a change in my weight even though I really "wanted" to lose. I quickly learned that just wanting it and actually making sacrifices to get there were two totally different things. The moment this really clicked for me was when I heard a man of God give the analogy of someone indicating he wanted to speak Spanish. He went on to explain the man didn't want to learn it, he just wanted to speak it. Now this really tickled me! It was just the visual I needed to identify my problem. There was a disconnect for me between wanting something and going after it.

Oftentimes we are like this with God. We want Him to do it or stop it or correct it. Sometimes He will, especially when we invite Him to take control over something and we totally surrender. On the other side of that coin, the "God just do it" mentality or genie in a bottle or even "miracle worker" for my church folks is not a demonstration of our commitment to Him or the process. And sometimes this expectation doesn't allow Him to work the "muscle" in us that is needed for many of the battles we will fight. Faith without works is dead! The more you work your faith muscle, the better you discern the route you must take.

You will know when God is telling you, His child to relax --- "Thus says the Lord to you: 'Do not be afraid nor dismayed because of this great multitude, for the battle is not yours, but God's.'" (2 Chronicles 20:15); and you will know when you are to conquer your challenge—"Yet in all these things we are more than conquerors through Him who loved us." (Romans 8:37).

You will trust when God says can take on your enemies—"For by You I can run against a troop, by my God I can leap over a wall." (Psalm 18:29) or when God does the impossible "But Jesus looked at them and said, 'With men it is impossible, but not with God; for with God all things are possible.'" (Mark 10:27).

Take it from my girls Mary Mary, in the amazing song *Go Get It, go get your blessing!* This is how your build your muscle. We must build both faith muscles and physical muscles! When a muscle isn't fully developed, it won't be able to perform in a way that will be fruitful. However, once it is developed, it grows and gets stronger.

In the Bible, when God had Joshua lead the new generation of Israelites into the Promised Land, He allowed them to conquer their enemies. This is how they received the land they were to inhabit. Yes, it was a land flowing with milk and honey, but other nations were there. Other tribes inhabited the land and they weren't going to just pick up and move. The children of Israel had to fight in order to receive God's promise to them and make their enemies move. Their parents on the other hand decided to murmur and complain and weren't able to receive the promise. Like Israel, will you be a complainer or a fighter?

On one occasion the descendants of Joseph came to Joshua saying they needed more land. They complained that they were too numerous for such a small amount of land. They made excuses and passed blame about the land allocated to them. I love Joshua's response. He didn't argue with them, or justify why they had received the specific land they were allotted; he didn't even tell them to deal with it and make do. His response was encompassed in a principle God had been trying to show His people all along.

He told them they could have more land in a particular area. Their excuse was they couldn't have that land because the Canaanites were there and they had iron chariots! Joshua's response to their lame excuse was amazing to me. He basically said, "Tell you what. Yes, you can have more land. There is plenty in the hill country and surrounding areas. You can have as much as you like. You told me you are too large for your current land, so I know you are strong and will be able to drive out the Canaanites. I believe in you! God get your Promised Land!"

"What? Coach, you want me to run three miles? Oh, but ten-pound weights are too heavy! I can't do that. I will stick to the five-pound weights because they are lighter. This meal plan is too hard for me—I want some French fries." Does any of this sound familiar? Has anything similar to that come out of your mouth before? Even when you don't feel like it or you don't feel like you can do it successfully, God is with you, guiding you out of your comfort zone. But, you have to fight to get your Promised Land!

God won't put an expectation on you that you aren't capable of fulfilling, the same way you wouldn't put an unrealistic expectation on your child. It doesn't make sense to have the expectation for your five-year-old to prepare dinner, right? However, you may have the expectation that at five he or she knows how to potty or put away the toys. Sounds silly, but we have to think about God as a good Father.

You've got this. You are God's child! I believe in you. You are stronger. Go, take the land you want." (Paraphrased) Yes! I believe in you! I believe you are God's kid and I believe that since you are reading this book, you can go take the land of your health and wellness. You can conquer the enemy who is telling you that you tried this before, or it is too hard, or you just don't feel like it today.

This is the great thing about inviting God in on this journey: The closer you stick to Him, the more confident you will be in defeating your enemies. God always wins and because you are made in His image, you should always win too! Woot Woot! Anything that comes between you and your health and fitness goals has to be crushed.

You Have to See It

Dream with God along this journey. Allow Him to ignite a vision in you to see yourself as He saw you even before time began. See yourself living a healthy life; see yourself going to the doctor in joy without a concern about a negative report. See yourself in those jeans or that bathing suit. Now, this is not an exercise of wishing you were skinny, whatever that means, but an exercise in seeing you living your best life in Christ, doing things you may not have been able to do before.

Once you see the dream and have the vision, partner your faith with God and work towards it. "Write the vision And make it plain on tablets, That he may run who reads it." (Habakkuk 2:2). Most of the time it will simply take you putting down your flesh and saying "NO" to your feelings. You dictate to them instead of them dictating to you. You will often have to use this word, especially with yourself. "No" to the extra servings because you see the vision. "No" to going out with the friends and indulging in things that are not going to get you to your goals. And "NO" to sitting on the couch and watching TV all night. "No, No, No!"

Do you realize that you, one person living your healthiest, whole life in Christ could change the world? Christ did! God sees all the seeds inside you, because the Greater One is inside of you. Sow these seeds into your health and you will be sowing seeds into communities, cities, countries, even continents.

I once read a book by Mike Murdock where he said, "The product of humility is the ability to change!" Now we can all stand more humility, but guess what, there is no change if there is no movement. Quitting doesn't speed up the process or get you any closer to your goals and the best life God has for you. It only ensures you won't get the prize. Your breakthrough is here but if you stop, you will never receive it! Make adjustments where you need to, not excuses.

Kicking Into Second Gear

Have you ever seen the movie *Overcomer*? If not, I highly recommend it. It's an amazing movie with an ending that may give itself away: someone overcomes. Haha! I will try not to spoil it for you, however there is a scene where a cross country runner is being coached through the championship run. Her coach tells her what to expect—her body will be exhausted; her legs will want to give out; that's when she will need to get her second wind and kick things into a higher gear! Huh? What? She's about to pass out and there is more? There is a higher level she can get to. There is more in you than you think there is. You are stronger than you know.

This is exactly what I'm sharing with you. When you want to quit, when you don't feel like going any further, that's the time that you will need to kick into higher gear. When you don't feel like it, listen to that inner voice, which is the Holy Spirit encouraging you to push through, to keep going, there is more in you! This may, however, indicate you are running on fumes. You may need to rest and recharge. Go to God, go back to your "whys" and remember the vision you had in the beginning. This is another attack of the enemy. But remember, he won't prevail.

Below are a few takeaways from Chapter Four. You may choose to come back and reflect on these later.

Lessons:

A. Having a "never give up attitude" will keep you successful on the journey. You will want to give up and will slip up for sure, but not staying in a defeated place gets you the victory.

B. Partner your faith with God for the vision He has given you. Hold on to that, keeping it in front of you for the rough times.

C. You will have to fight for what you want and what might rightfully belong to you. Get off the "trying" wheel and get at it. It will require you saying NO to people and Your flesh man.

Confessions:

- Blessed be the Lord my Rock, Who trains my hands for war and my fingers for battle. (Psalm 144:1).

- Now thanks be to God who always leads me in triumph in Christ, and through me diffuses the fragrance of His knowledge in every place. (2 Corinthians 2:14).

- I can do all things through Christ who strengthens me. (Philippians 4:13).

- For by You I can run against a troop, By my God I can leap over a wall. (Psalm 18:29).

- I am hard-pressed on every side, yet not crushed; I am perplexed, but not in despair; persecuted, but not forsaken; struck down, but not destroyed. (2 Corinthians 4:8).

Prayer:

Father,

Help me to see the vision, but not only to see the vision, to fight for it to come to pass, to continue in a forward motion even when I don't feel like. I choose to no longer live in the excuse zone. I choose to no longer allow my feelings and emotions to control and rule me. I will acknowledge where I have not done my part, quickly repent and reset. I ask that you would teach my hands to war and my fingers to fight. I am resilient, I am victorious in this battle and I refuse to be defeated because I belong to you! I declare and decree this now in Jesus Mighty Name I pray! Amen

CHAPTER FIVE

WHEN YOU FALL DOWN

<u>The Road Won't Be Easy</u>

T o be perfectly honest, there will be challenges, but you can't let them define you or stop you from moving forward. You have to remain steadfast in your determination and consistent in your commitment. Consistency leads to lasting change. This is how you build your habit muscles. This is why all of our programs at Kingdom Power Living are built upon consistency and accountability. Notice the title of this chapter isn't *if* you fall down, it's *when* you fall down, because everyone falls down, myself included.

The focus is not about the falling down though. What's more important is the getting back up. The Bible is clear that when the righteous fall seven times they get back up. "For a righteous man may fall seven times And rise again, But the wicked shall fall by calamity." (Proverbs 24:16). Is that you? Are you the righteous one being described in this scripture? Well then, be sure to get back up. One way to help when you fall down is to get up quickly. Having accountability systems in place will help too.

Falling Doesn't Equal Failure

We are not often told when growing up we are going to fail. Perhaps that is a good thing because who really wants to hear such a word of discouragement? However, maybe we need to redefine what failure is. Falling doesn't equal failure. According to the Word of God the righteous may fall seven times but get back up. Even Paul said in Romans that he didn't do the very things he wanted to do, but did the things that he didn't want to do. "For what I am doing, I do not understand. For what I will to do, that I do not practice; but what I hate, that I do." (Romans 7:15). It won't always be easy. You won't always make the right decisions but that's okay if you get back up and get back in the game. I tell my clients and even practice myself, "Reset quickly!"

There is a call on your life. The enemy will try to get you to take your eyes off the vision because the vision is God's plan for you. Once you believe that, you will be dangerous to the enemy and victorious for the kingdom.

There is absolutely warfare against your health and wellness, but you have to be smart, strategic and determined in this important area. Who wants to work out anyway, right? You are targeted because of the dream and the vision inside you. You may be targeted with shame, with doubt, with fear, with guilt, with unbelief and so on because of what is yet to be birthed inside you. God designed plans and a purpose for you even before you were created. Jesus is advocating for you and when you are weak, He is strong. "And He said to me, 'My grace is sufficient for you, for My strength is made perfect in weakness.'" (2 Corinthians 12:9). So, don't stop! Keep going.

I remember when one of my clients was restricting certain foods in her diet, like refined processed carbohydrates. She was still cooking regularly for the family, who were not eating the same meal plan. I do recommend getting the entire family on board eating the same healthy meals if possible, however, I know that can be a challenge—but flow with me.

In the process of preparing dinner, which this night was pasta, she tasted one of the noodles to see if it was cooked through—unconsciously, because this was what she always did when preparing pasta. However, since she wasn't eating pasta at the time, she immediately when into a place of failure and set back. She beat herself up for having that one pasta noodle and thought her whole plan was thrown off because of it.

Not so! Nothing could be further from the truth. I assured her that her goals were still on track and she would be fine. This one derailment could have caused her to spiral down a rabbit hole like many of us have experienced unnecessarily. Even if the diet was hit, guess what—get back up and start again! It's never over if you still have breath in your body. It's important to recognize the voice of the enemy when he is trying to beat you up and condemn you. That is never the Father's heart, so recognize the counterfeit and keep moving along.

The enemy will try to make you focus on the fall so you lose sight of the bigger picture and the dream God has for you, your life and the lives of others. The enemy will try to shame you into disbelieving the big purpose of God. Condemnation leads to shame, but conviction leads to change. Always remember that. If you are feeling shame for falling or getting off track, know it isn't God and it isn't His plan for you to stay there. Jump off that burning train as soon as possible, before you get seriously injured.

It may sound a little ridiculous to some but this is exactly the game the enemy plays, making us feel like its worthless and we have messed up beyond repair. The lie will then snowball into, "See, I told you you couldn't do this healthy eating thing, you messed up, you are right back where you started, you're a failure, you couldn't even do this." And so on and so on. I'm telling you this because I have been there. This is when you go back to your identity.

God is the God of the mountain top as well as the valley low. We cannot and should no stay in the valley. We don't go from mountain top to mountain top. In the same way, we don't go from valley to valley. There are seasons and there are victories in every season, even in the midst of tough times. "For His anger is but for a moment, His favor is for life; Weeping may endure for a night, but joy comes in the morning." (Psalm 30:5) Have your short period of weeping and then bounce back to joy quickly in the morning! You've got this!

Memories of past failures are sure to haunt you. Emotions of hopelessness or insecurity will creep in, but you were built for this. I read somewhere that the acronym for F.A.I.L. is "first attempt in learning." I don't think that falling down, especially the falling down the Bible speaks of, is synonymous with failure. However, what I do like about the acronym is its suggestion that you don't stay there at that place. One of my favorite speakers says it something like this: "Failure only occurs when you don't get back up, not when you fall down." So, like in boxing, if I can use another sports analogy, as long as you keep getting back up, the fight continues.

Sure, you may have not been as successful as you would have liked with some of your past diet or exercise attempts, but that was just part of the learning process. However, when you do this with God as the foundation, He is the solid rock that winds and rain can beat against and it will still stand! Make the decision to get back up and not go back as Israel Houghton declares in his song *Moving Forward*. Make a decision over and over again to move forward, no matter the cost. Declare that your past is over. In Christ you are a new creation. You are not your past!

Do you know how many people attempted something before the actual realization came to life? Thomas Edison, made one thousand attempts at inventing the light bulb before he finally got to the winner. A reporter allegedly asked how he felt failing one thousand times and, his response was "I didn't fail one thousand times. The light bulb was an invention with one thousand steps." Michael Jordan was cut from his high school basketball team. Abraham Lincoln went to war as a captain, and came back a private. He failed in business and failed many times running for several political office before becoming the president. Einstein was thought to be behind developmentally as he didn't speak until he was four years old and didn't read until he was seven years old. Sidney Poitier was told by a casting director, "Why don't you stop wasting people's time and go out and become a dishwasher or something?" Marilyn Monroe, who isn't typically portrayed as the size she really was, (in the 12-14 size range) was told by a director to go and get married or do secretarial work.

This hopefully paints a picture for you, that no matter how you start, it is always about how you finish. The lesson here isn't that it's okay to keep falling. Well, maybe it is or maybe it is how we look at and learn from falling, how we look at setbacks in order to step forward; how we don't give up. Please don't take this as confirmation that yoyo dieting is okay or normal. And it's definitely not for you look at the past and say, "See it didn't work then, therefore it won't work now." In every one of the above examples, famous people that you know and may admire kept at it. They continued taking multiple attempts until reaching greatness, it could have been easy for them to stop at any point and say, "It's not working." But they didn't! They kept moving forward and so will you! There are many more examples, but hopefully this is enough of a taste for you to understand where I'm coming from. You are always moving either forward or backward. There is no middle ground. Keep pushing, you've got this!

Find Your Momentum

It's kind of like "Stay in your lane and crush it!" Clients come to me with eating plans they have tried—low carb, keto, whole 30, Atkins, low fat, and so on, and so on. There are so many schools of thought and diverse opinions on all of these diets. Many argue that cutting out whole food groups is a problem or consuming too much of something is a problem.

While I believe there could be benefits to any of them, what we need to hone in on is what works best for you. I don't believe in a one-size-fits-all approach. What can you commit to as a lifestyle is the question I always ask? You see celebrities promote certain plans. You watch YouTube channels and scan the internet for others that are the latest trend and you want to buy into that. Many of these plans have given people extremely good results but going on another diet will not be the key to your success. There is no short cut. You will have to put in the work, consistently and continuously. This requires a mindset shift for a lifestyle change.

I am all about fueling your body — and that should be done for the rest of your life. So, find what works for you, find your momentum and stick with it! Whatever it is, it shouldn't put or keep you in any sort of bondage. That's not God's best for you and your best is always His goal. When you glorify Him in your body, you are living in His best for you!

Oh, but I do understand and can relate to that fear of failure. I have dealt with it most of my childhood and some of my adult life. In junior high I played on the volleyball team at our small Catholic school. I was okay. I had a good underhand serve that kept me coming back. Our team wasn't great and we didn't go very far, but it was fun and I enjoyed it.

Once I got to high school that desire to play volleyball was still in me but there was also a little voice inside that said, "You know you aren't that good. This is a completely different level and these girls have been playing together since elementary. They have the skills, they know each other, your thighs are too big for those little shorts they wear, they don't look like you and you know you just don't fit in. You probably won't make the team, so don't even try out."

That entire narrative played out in my head more than once. I can even hear it so clearly today. Guess what I didn't do? I didn't try out for the team. My home period teacher was the volleyball coach. Hello! And I allowed a fear of failure to stop me from even trying. But what if I had just tried? I may have been an Olympic volleyball player—or not. I may have tried it and figured out quickly, this isn't the sport for me. However, because I didn't even try, I will never know. God can bring redemption. That is why we invite Him on the journey, but my point here is we can't let fear stop us from trying.

Now, years later, I have a choice, I can either sit here and play the "what if" game or choose to live in the present. Stepping out even when we are afraid rids us of playing the "what if" game. We will know! We will know if it works out or not and move accordingly. Now, there is some danger in continuing to sit around year after year and wondering, "What if?" You have to move on. You have to let it go, renew your mind and not let your past torment you forever.

It still tries to creep up every now and again, like when you hear, "Write a book." The constant struggle returns—what if this doesn't work, what if people don't like it, what if you lose, what if you go back to the same way you were before? What if, what if, what if? And my response usually is "What if you don't?" There are always two sides to every coin. Yes, there are chances it won't work, but there are also chances it will and the odds are probably better on this side, because God is with you!

Now, if you are somewhat risk-averse like me, you may feel like you don't want to take the chance. However, I believe the stakes are too high for you not to. Way out, what is the worst that can happen? You actually believe God and get your life back or you stay where you are in an unhappy, unhealthy place? That doesn't sound like abundant life. Even if you have set-backs, there are always lessons to be learned. I'm sure you have heard the saying that the set back "didn't happen to you, it happened for you." There are always lessons to be learned. Inventions and prototypes go through many iterations before releasing the final product. Evaluate the setback, see what God wants you to learn from it and then open those wings and begin to fly again!

<u>Never Give Up</u>

A couple of years ago when I was still working in corporate America, I had to go to the UK for work. I had never been there before, so I was excited. It was a whirlwind of a trip. We hit three countries in less than a week. We traveled by planes, trains, buses and automobiles. It was quite exhausting, with the last leg of the trip landing us in London. After our last meeting, we had the opportunity to just chill and enjoy the city for the next two days. It became pretty clear that my colleague had plans of her own, which quickly became okay with me because I'm used to rolling solo.

I soon came up with the bright idea to travel to Paris for the day. I had never been there and I had heard so many people talking about how amazing it was. This was my shot, so I began to look into what this adventure might look like even though I was a little nervous. It didn't seem real. I prayed about it and asked God to show me and make it clear if it was okay to go on this adventure.

I try to use wisdom as much as possible, being a woman traveling on my own. I found the best route. It was only a train ride away. Ticket prices weren't so bad but I didn't move right away and they soon spiked. This made me not want to go, but the weather in London was going to be awful the next day so I thought I would rather be in Paris than rainy and cold in London. I bought the more expensive tickets and set off the next morning.

I will spare you all of the details of what happened in Paris. I will tell you three things though. First, I didn't like Paris at all. Second, I did get my delicious street crêpe. And third, I missed my train back to London, the very last train of the night! And I was due to leave early the next morning to return home! Paris time was ahead of London's and for some reason my clock did not automatically reset to the new time zone.

At first, I thought it was a joke when the gentleman at the train station told me the train back to London had already departed. Then I realized that it wasn't a joke but a very bad dream. I was devastated. My mind quickly began to go into defense mode! I had to fix this. I had to figure out a way to get back to London, even though it didn't look promising.

This is what I need from you. I need your brain to quickly begin to think of ways to get back home with your health. Don't stay too long in the place of "I missed my train, I ate two donuts, I'm such a loser, what's wrong with me, I messed up, I should have never…" This is the time where you quickly fix the problem.

It is okay to go back and analyze what went wrong in order to prevent it from happening again. It is okay also to just repent and move on. This is another example where the enemy will try to creep in and bring condemnation, shame and guilt, trying to make you torture yourself and stay in a stuck place. This is never God's heart.

The reason my brain immediately went to "fix it" mode is partially because that's how God wired me as a problem solver and partially because I am a fighter and never give up. You are a fighter too and can never give up!

That day in Paris felt like one of the biggest mistakes of my life. How could I have gotten myself into this? Did I not hear the voice of the Holy Spirit? Was I just in the flesh? Or was this part of God's plan to build upon a resilience muscle that needed a little more work?

It could have been a combination of all of the above. Although that time in Paris was awful, again, I will spare you all the details of the tears, the rejection, the all-night travel back to London that carried over into the morning, and the pretty-much-straight-to-the-airport trip with a quick detour to my hotel room to grab my luggage! It brought to life the scripture that He works all things together for my good. "And we know that all things work together for good to those who love God, to those who are the called according to His purpose." (Romans 8:28).

That was me; that was what I was standing on through the entire process. That is you too, that is what I want you to stand on. It doesn't matter about the past, the past attempts, the past hurts, the past self-sabotages. He works all things together for your good! It's a promise you can stand on, it's His promise to you. And I want you to promise me that you will never give up. No matter the past, it's a new day and a new season!

Accountability is Key

Accountability is very important on this journey. However, it puts you in a vulnerable state and not everyone will ask for it or welcome it. Having a system helps at times when you just don't want to do it. For example, if a friend checks on you for not going to the gym, welcome that feedback, because you have given that person permission to speak into your life. My clients know that I am going to hold them accountable. If you don't want that, don't give me that authority, don't sign up for my programs, and don't ask for my help because you really just want to do what you want to do.

I recently heard a saying. "Being interested in a particular thing only when it is convenient is not being committed to it." Therefore, convenience doesn't equal commitment. It is like casual dating, you are not committed, you are simply enjoying yourself while it is good. You could be interested in a pair of $1,000 Louboutin shoes, but you are not committed until you dish out the cash to purchase them. Commitment is when you pursue results until you get them, without making excuses. Commitment must be your focus and not a casual interest for lasting transformation. If you fall down, that's okay. Just get up and do it again. Learn from your falls so your future accountability can be more effective.

We have discussed that not everyone will be in your corner on this journey and that is okay. However, it is important to have accountability in place. This may come in the form of a tribe or it may be reminders and systems you set in place. For instance, one system may be scheduling your workouts on your calendar like you do other important, non-negotiable meetings and appointments. Workouts fit in the same category as one-on-one meetings with your manager, or doctor's appointments, or date nights with your spouse. You don't want to cancel those.

Another option is you may choose is to have a workout partner with whom you exercise or go to the gym together; or you may just have the person who sends you a text and checks in to make sure you are still going strong. Whatever works for you is fine. The important piece is to be honest with yourself about what really works for you and what you are really willing to commit to. If not, this won't work!

If you do have a tribe supporting you, great. However, don't get this group confused with the "yes" crowd. Your tribe is comprised of those who will support you and help pick you back up when you fall. You also give them permission to get in your face and tell you when you are wrong, when you are off course, when you are not fighting, and when you are not living up to your full potential. This person or group of people will not let you give up!

Below are a few takeaways from Chapter Five. You may choose to come back and reflect on these later.

Lessons:

A. The road won't be perfect, smooth or easy, however, with the proper accountability systems and commitment you can conquer it.

B. You are not a failure even when you fall down. Your success is in getting back up. When you focus too long on what happened, you begin to stay in that place. Learn quickly and move on.

C. How you finish is more important than how you start. Find your groove and keep up the momentum. This is where the lifestyle change occurs and lasts.

<u>Confessions:</u>

- That He would grant me, according to the riches of His glory, to be strengthened with might through His Spirit in my inner man. (Ephesians 3:16).

- Yet in all these things I am more than a conqueror through Him who loved me. (Romans 8:37).

- And I overcame him by the blood of the Lamb and by the word of my testimony, and I do not love my life to the death. (Revelation 12:11).

- For a righteous man may fall seven times And rise again... (Proverbs 24:16).

Prayer:

Father,

In the Name of Jesus, I am not a failure even though I may fall sometimes. I will learn from every mistake and determine not to stay down. I am more than a conqueror because the Greater One lives inside of me! I will set up and use the accountability systems you give me. I ask you to bring me the right resources and tribe according to your will. Ultimately I know that I am not in this alone since I have invited you on the journey. I repent for the times I didn't come to you but operated in my own strength. I know I need your wisdom and your strength and I will pay whatever price necessary! My heart is for you to get the glory in all of this! Use me Lord even through my mess ups and mistakes. In Jesus Name I Pray! Amen.

CHAPTER SIX

WHERE IS YOUR IDENTITY?

Identification Card Please

Everything boils down to this. Your health, wellness and fitness journey will continue to go forth as you continue to remember who you are in Christ. The first step was making the decision, the second step was renewing your mind, followed by commitment, goals, etc. But your identity is what's going to keep you soaring along the journey. Similar to your "whys," knowing who you are causes you to walk in who God created you, keep focused and move forward.

The gospel singer Sinach sings a song that I really like—*I know who I am*. When you know who you are, no one and nothing can stop you. Period. Well, except maybe you! But when that happens, you are still not believing what God has said about you and you are sabotaging yourself. You have to know who you are on this journey. I can't stress that enough. Anything less than that will keep you on the cycle of up-and-down weight loss and dieting or just a constant state of doing nothing, believing the lie that you aren't ready. You are always positioned to be ready, even if you are seemingly not ready, so do it while you aren't ready! God has you. He won't leave you even when you fall.

Royalty Acts Like Royalty

I love it when my clients can be themselves. I know they love it too—they tell me so. Free to be exactly who God created you to be, no masks, no perfection, true authenticity and embracing the wonderfulness that God created in you! When you feel like you have to put on a face for others, do you really know who God says you are? No, you are trying to be acceptable in the eyes of others because you have not yet discovered your royalty. Since we are talking about soaring. Have you ever noticed how regal an eagle is? They are swift, powerful and revered. And so are you!

One of my favorite scriptures in the Bible is James 1. It encourages us not to look in the mirror of God's Word, then immediately forget who we are. "For if anyone is a hearer of the word and not a doer, he is like a man observing his natural face in a mirror; for he observes himself, goes away, and immediately forgets what kind of man he was." (James 1:23-24). Once you have really grasped your identity in Christ, the things that were once temptations, setbacks or roadblocks will no longer be, because your identity reminds you that the Greater One lives inside of you!

No longer can you live in shame or guilt or unforgiveness or pride or any of those things, because of your identity. No longer can you see yourself as the overweight person who is helpless and can't change. No longer can you continue to tell yourself you are not ready, or continue to hide in the shadows because you don't know your identity and are afraid to come forth. No longer do you identify as the person with the eating disorder who doesn't like to look in the mirror, because now when you look in the mirror you see the image of God! The old has passed away and you are new. "Therefore, if anyone is in Christ, he is a new creation; old things have passed away; behold, all things have become new." (2 Corinthians 5:17) This is not who you are anymore. You are now the new you!

The Father's Touch

This reminds me of a time when I was taking a walk in my neighborhood. There was a sweet little girl riding her bike. It was obvious that her ride was a little shaky, which explained the strong but gentle man who stood close by just in case she needed some support. And sure enough she did. The sweet little girl began to wobble and lean, ever so slightly to the left. In this instant, the strong but gentle man by her side simply positioned his hip ever so slightly to the right against the girl and her bike and wrapped his arm around her. She paused momentarily and then started back on her way with the strong but gentle man still by her side.

It was the most precious thing I had seen in a long time. It was exactly what I needed, as God gently spoke to me and reassured me that He was there to catch me when and if I fall. He is there to catch you as well.

The Father's gentle touch and His constant presence confirm your identity as His child. He will be there with you if you even begin to fall. But you have to know who you are in Him—His child. That is your identity! Believe it! So that when times get rough, because they will get rough, look up and remember again and again. It will take constant renewing of the mind to win.

Slightly off topic, but still related. When I knew who I was and that God had a great plan for marriage, I wasn't tempted by dating or trying to find someone to date. My identity as a woman of God was greater than my desire to have a temporary emotional feeling that could easily slip by if it wasn't God's will for my life. Seeing myself as the bride of Christ allowed me to be content whether married or not, because I knew who and whose I was. Once you really grasp that concept, the negative habits and behaviors cannot keep you bound.

On the flip side, you need to see yourself as healthy and whole. Identify yourself as the person who is making healthy choices and buying healthy food that fuels your body; as the person who now works out multiple times a week; the person who now bench presses heavy weights instead of the person who makes heavy or fat jokes to try to hide the pain.

God has a good reason for instructing us to be ready and equipped in His armor, ready to fight the enemy. We are going to have to fight; there is no way around it. "Put on the whole armor of God, that you may be able to stand against the wiles of the devil." (Ephesians 6:11) If you have your armor on, the old lies and fiery darts are not able to penetrate. They fall to the ground, having no effect and you continue to operate like the soldier you were created to be! Right? Now that's good and something to do your happy dance about.

Comparison Will Kill You

Don't look around at others and wonder, "What if?" Nobody can do you the way that you do you! Nobody has the same DNA, make up or even body composition. There may be similarities, but no one is like you. You are unique, you are distinctive, and you are rare like a precious jewel. When you begin to look at others and compare yourself to them, you forget the beauty of who you are.

The spleen doesn't compare itself to the eye and the leg doesn't compare itself to the liver. How silly would it be if the leg said to the liver, "I like the way you are shaped. I wish I was your size. I wish I could flush toxins out but instead all I can do is carry weight and help the body move." Okay, a little exaggerated, but doesn't that sound ridiculous? Well, that's exactly what we are doing when we compare ourselves to others.

One of the ways this manifests is not taking care of our temples. You either put pressure on yourself to be something that isn't possible or you escape and hide, not maintaining the soil you are appointed to tend. God created you and knows the number of hairs you have on your head. Not everyone has the same number of hairs on their head. This is a big deal, because He not only knows yours, but He knows mine and Kim's and Sarah's and Felicia's and Tiffany's!

Ask the Lord to heal you of every lie that has been spoken to you, about you and over you, especially from your past. Begin to break every curse and chain of defeat over your life, particularly in the area of your fitness, health and wellness, a space that probably has been left dormant for a while, a place unattended and wide open for the attacks of the enemy. Trade every lie for His truth. Declare "No more!" Today we end this and soar above the old way of seeing ourselves! Spend time with God in this season and beyond, listening to and learning from Him, knowing your true identity in Him. Begin to see what He sees: perfection made by the work of His hands!

He never gives up on you, even when you give up on yourself. Even when others around you, those closest to you, may give up, He never will. "When my father and my mother forsake me, Then the Lord will take care of me." (Psalm 27:10). Really, get this inside your heart and rehearse this narrative in your mind. The Bible says God wants all to be saved. Some choose to leave but that is not what He wants.

Be comfortable with being the real you He designed before the foundations of the world. Be willing to be different. Be the leader others want to follow. Be comfortable with being the family member who doesn't eat or indulge in the same bad habits as others. Become comfortable with saying "no." Become comfortable with bringing your own food if necessary. Be comfortable putting your flesh down and letting your Spirit man rule.

I know that may sound a bit extreme and a little over-the-top, but why can't we be that way as temples of the Holy Spirit? God has told us to glorify Him in in our bodies. Are you willing to be that extreme and radical with your faith and fitness? This has to be the new normal, so get used to it and enjoy!

Below are a few takeaways from Chapter Six. You may choose to come back and reflect on these later.

Lessons:

A. See and believe that you are not who you used to be, no matter what anyone says to you or tells you along the way. Accepting Christ means that old person is dead.

B. Royalty acts like royalty. When you really know who you are in Christ, you won't go back to the same destructive, self-sabotaging behaviors. You will be free.

C. When you are comfortable being who God truly created you to be, you will see how pointless it is to compare yourself to others.

Confessions:

- …as I have received Him, He gave me the right to become a child of God, to me who believes in His name. (John 1:12).

- But I am a chosen generation, a royal priesthood, a holy nation, His own special people, that I may proclaim the praises of Him who called me out of darkness into His marvelous light. (1 Peter 2:9).

- He has made everything beautiful in its time. (Ecclesiastes 3:11).

- I believe in You, the works that You do I will do also; and greater works than these I will do, because You went to The Father. (John 14:12).

- I abide in You, and You in me. As the branch cannot bear fruit of itself, unless it abides in the vine, neither can I, unless I abide in You. (John 15:4).

- And because I am a son, God has sent forth the Spirit of His Son into my heart, crying out, "Abba, Father!" (Galatians 4:6).

Prayer:

Father,

I know my identity should be in you. But more than just knowing this, I want to live it. I don't want to ever forget who I am in you. I am a child of God and I am determined live like this every day, even on the rough days, even when it's hard and things are not going so well. In the valleys and on the mountain tops I want to continue to see myself as you see me. I will behave as the royal priesthood that you designed me to be. I will not compare myself to others or envy others' walks or accomplishments. I will remain steadfast in you and fight for every breakthrough. Thank you for your touch and being here every step of the way on this journey. I am not alone and I am proud to bear the name of God's child. No weapon formed against me shall prosper. In Jesus Name I pray! Amen.

CHAPTER SEVEN

YOU HAVE THE VICTORY

Believe It's For You

My prayer now is that you believe this newness of life, this kingdom lifestyle, is for you! Believe that this change is for you, it belongs to you and you deserve it. As long as you accept the lie of the enemy, defeat will knock on your door. Remember and go back to:

- Making a Decision
- Mind Renewal
- Identity and
- Worth

Whenever you feel insecure on this journey, look back to the cross, the ultimate sign of your victory.

I remember when I was recommended to interview Mellody Hobson. Those who are Chicago natives may be familiar with her, and for any *Star Wars* fans, she is the wife of George Lucas.

I was still working in corporate America during that time and co-chaired our women's group for the firm. We wanted to get a big name for our women's history month event and I asked any senior leader who would listen if we could get her. She was on our Board and probably the biggest female name in investment banking.

Once it looked like we were going to get her, the next logical thing to do was to think about was who would interview her. Someone in the room mentioned my name. This shocked me: one, because I didn't know the person who recommended me thought highly of me; and two, because I felt insecure about who I was. I didn't have a high enough position or title to interview someone with such great accomplishments. You see, I had listened to the lie of the enemy.

I short-changed myself and didn't believe it was for me because I didn't recognize the victory God had placed within me. I wasn't believing the scripture "I can do all things through Christ who strengthens me." (Philippians 4:13). I was looking at outward circumstances, the past and limiting beliefs instead of the Word of God. This is what I want to communicate to you! You too have the victory as long as you look to Him and not to yourself. The sky is the limit on things you can accomplish through Him because you already have the victory!

You were created to change people's lives. This may or may not mean millions around the world. However, it definitely means the short-list around you, those within arm's reach, those who need you to be the healthiest, most whole you possible.

<u>Victory Belongs to You</u>

In closing, I want to encourage you to keep your mind stayed on Him. Focus on the things above and not on circumstances around you which can change. "If then you were raised with Christ, seek those things which are above, where Christ is, sitting at the right hand of God. Set your mind on things above, not on things on the earth." (Colossians 3:1-2).

Don't focus on shortcomings or obstacles you encounter because if you have read the end of the Book, you know you ultimately win. If you keep this in front of you, there is nothing you won't be able accomplish. Remember, with God, nothing shall be impossible. If you are with God, all things are possible!

The day I first stepped into a Nike fitness class, I was scared! I thought of every excuse not to go. The limiting beliefs were running through my head faster than a fifty-five-meter sprint. What if they looked at me in a way that rejected me? My thoughts raced: "I'm sure all the other ladies will be so much more athletic than me; the instructor may wonder why am I here; I may not be able to complete the workout; what if they will find out how weak I really am; I can't even do a full push up..." I mean, every excuse under the sun tried to prevent me seeing how strong I really was. Even if everything I thought were true, continuing to go through with the workout showed the enemy my thoughts were not the boss of me and I wasn't going to stay stuck in the position I was in. I made the decision to take the first step. I had to fight through all the noise and go back to my "why" in Christ. And it all worked out! Look at me now!

What did He say about me? Even if all those things in my mind were true, they couldn't define me because God already had. He said something different from my feelings. If they did look at me in a strange way, so what! I could look back with a smile. So what if I couldn't finish the exercises? I tried! What if the instructor did wonder why I was there? Maybe I was wondering why the instructor was teaching the class! Lol My point is none of that mattered.

Sometimes it's the enemy, sometimes it's you, and sometimes it's all about perspective. You do in either case choose whether to believe the lie or not. Even if the situation happened in a manner you dreaded, it didn't kill you! You learned a lesson and now you can pass the test on that lesson, move on and help others in the future with the same or a similar challenge.

Sometimes it is just a part of the test. The whole point of the test is to show and prove that you know the information you have been taught or the area you have been trained in. When you follow your dream, you will be met with opposition, but this can't stop you! Why? Because God has already declared you have the victory! Doing it relationally with God is the whole goal, and for sure the game changer. Have you got the message yet? God has already given you the victory! I have said it over and over again because I really want this to get into your heart and into your spirit—you have the victory! There it goes again! I'm going to leave you with yet another song as we wrap things up. It's Tye Tribbett's *Victory*. Now, I want you to crank this one all the way up! Go right now and get your dance on again because you truly do have the V.I.C.T.O.R.Y!

Practical Tips

If you are just starting out, start where you are. There is no rush for this because this is your lifestyle now, your new normal. You are not on a diet or quick trick weight loss plan. You have made the decision to invite God on this journey. It's a marathon, not a sprint. The goal is to glorify Him all along the way. This isn't temporal. This is a process you have embraced. It is now your life's mission because you too have others to impact.

If you are haven't moved in a while, start with a walk for as long as you can. Remember, baby steps are still steps! Begin to challenge yourself and go higher from there. If you start with a five-minute walk, next week try to go to seven or ten and up from there.

If you start with two or more days of exercising, pace yourself. Listen to how your body feels. Consider taking a break in between days and establish them as your rest and recover days.

You will feel some soreness—I still feel soreness—push through as much as possible. However, recovery needed, so be sure to incorporate recovery days. Just don't break for too long.

Everyone Loves a Good Fight

There was a time when we moved to a new neighborhood. I didn't know many people except my cousins. We lived together and they were with me. We walked to the nearby store, probably for some snacks, I can't remember now. What I do remember was encountering a few boys who weren't so welcoming to our new faces.

Before I knew it, I was in a fight that I didn't invite, nor did I enjoy, especially fighting a boy! But I knew what I had to do. I gave it everything I had and then something happened... I was dominating the scene. I had not only given this boy a run for his money, I was winning! I've always had some fight in me.

Others standing around witnessed my victory. As a proud champ with a small weight title under my belt, I began to walk off and continue minding my business, only to quickly discover he had a twin brother who then tried to switch shirts and pretend he was the first brother, and fight me. I guess he knew it wasn't right to double-team a girl, but he still wanted to defend his brother's honor and fight a girl. Go figure!

At this point, it wasn't necessary for me to continue with the shenanigans. I knew who I was, I knew I had won, I knew I already had the victory and I didn't have to continue in another fight at that time just to prove it. Do you see where I'm going here? I knew who I was, so I didn't have to continue with the enemy's plan and try to prove something. You too have the victory. It's yours! Know who you are in the fight—the victor, not the victim!!!

Progress Over Perfection

I'm sure you have heard the saying "progress over perfection." It undertake is so true and I need you to do more than give this a fleeting thought. Incorporate it as a principle to live by on this journey. Thinking you have to be perfect, or this journey must be perfect, is many times rooted in fear. It will never be perfect and you waiting for perfection stops progress.

Progress depicts forward movement. It won't always look pretty, trust me. When you wait for perfection, it becomes a waiting game and you are not moving forward. Movement is definitely the name of the game you are playing. So, accept right now that every day won't be great or easy, and be okay with that as long as you are moving forward! Remember the Israel Houghton song?

When God called Lot and his family out of Sodom and Gomorrah, He instructed them not to look back but to keep moving ahead out of the land. Lot's wife looked back and turned into a pillar of salt. Determine never to give up or look back!

Be certain to track your progress because we at Kingdom Power Living celebrate all victories, big and small. When you go from that five-minute walk to that seven-minute walk, get excited and celebrate. When you lose two pounds, celebrate. When you can now fit the jeans that have been in the back of your closet for three years, celebrate.

Record God's goodness in getting you there as a praise report or memorial as the Israelites did, creating memorials to mark and remember God's faithfulness! This showed their enemies or haters who their God really was. Show off your God to your haters. Show off His goodness to you along this journey. The world needs to see and hear. It's awesome to beat the devil's head in when he challenges you to return to old ways but you choose forward progress, even small progress. Remember, reverting is not us anymore.

Most of my programs come with a prayer pad so that you can jot down your prayers along the way. Record your prayer requests to God, have supporting scriptures to stand on, and celebrate testimonies when those prayers get answered. That's like the children of Israel with the memorial. It also encourages and strengthens your faith. I believe it is pleasing to God because He gets the glory! And He is not going to share His glory with anyone! "...no flesh should glory in His presence." (1 Corinthians 1:29).

Now is the time to write your story. You have the ability to produce the outcome you want. It's not too late! Because you have made it to the last chapter, you have everything needed to keep going and live the kingdom life you deserve. With you and Christ on this journey, nothing is impossible. It's your time to soar higher and higher.

Below are a few takeaways from Chapter Seven. You may choose to come back and reflect on these later.

Lessons:

A. It is okay to step out because God has already given you the victory no matter how difficult or uncomfortable. You win either way!

B. Victory doesn't mean you did it perfectly. It means you have adopted a new kingdom lifestyle, where you are living your best, healthiest life for Christ—not in perfection, but progressively each day.

C. Celebrate every win, no matter how small or how big. Every time you conquer something, write it down as a memorial. Honor every victory and treat it as royal, just like you!

Confessions:

- I am born of God; I overcome the world. And this is the victory that has overcome the world—my faith. (1 John 5:4).

- But thanks be to God, who gives me the victory through my Lord Jesus Christ. (1 Corinthians 15:57).

- A bruised reed He will not break, And smoking flax He will not quench, Till He sends forth justice to victory. (Matthew 12:20).

- You have also given me the shield of Your salvation; Your right hand has held me up, Your gentleness has made me great. (Psalm 18:35).

- So I may boldly say: "The LORD is my helper; I will not fear. What can man do to me?" (Hebrews 13:6).

Prayer:

Father,

Thank you for the victory I have you. In YOU I live, in YOU I move and in YOU I have my being. I will no longer try to be a perfectionist but continue progressing in you. I will celebrate every win and see it as victory. I will no longer operate in fear because YOU have given me the Spirit of love, the Spirit of power and a sound mind. I believe and confess that the victory does belong to me, not because of anything I have done in and of myself, but because of YOU. Thank you for everything you have done and will continue to do in me. Thank you for working and willing in me to do of your good pleasure. Thank you for not loosening your grip on me, and thank you for making me a part of your very own family. I am delighted to know that I can do all things through Christ who strengthens me and that nothing is impossible with you. Without faith it is impossible to please God, so I will continue to lean on my faith to live the very best kingdom lifestyle, knowing that I am pleasing to you, my Father in Heaven. In Jesus Name I pray! Amen.

CHAPTER EIGHT

WHAT NOW?

Next Steps

Okay, so if you are at this part of the book, you are probably wondering or asking me if you were across from me, "What's next?" I've gotten you all fired up with all the foundational stuff and now it is time to implement, implement, implement.

If I were to give you three things to kickstart the fitness journey, because we have talked a lot about the faith, I would say:

1. Increase your water intake now! Go get a bottle of water right now and drink it all.
2. Remove white table sugar from your diet and eat as clean as possible. What I mean by "clean" is eating foods with the least amount of processing and are as natural as possible.
3. Get your body moving now!

Let's start with the water. When you were growing up, I'm sure your doctor or mom or someone told you to drink eight glasses of water each day. Those glasses were probably eight ounces which makes for sixty-four ounces. In today's world, that would be roughly four plastic water bottles that you get from the store, slightly more as many are 16.9 ounces. That is great! Most people aren't doing that.

However, there is a new-school way of thinking that says water is way too important for the body, and it is recommended for you to consume up to half your body weight in ounces of water. Now, you are probably saying, "What! No way can I drink that much water." I am here to challenge you that you certainly can! There are healthy ways to get this amount of water in, as well as various apps out there that will help you track your water intake.

Like everything else we have discussed in this book, it takes dedication and commitment to make this happen, including a little bit of planning.

We can take it even further, which I do in some of my courses and challenges, to drink up to a gallon of water each day. Again, you can do this safely. There are so many benefits to water, including hydration, flushing out toxins from your body, boosting your metabolism and so on.

This will require you to use the rest room often, but you will normalize. You can and should stop your intake a couple hours before bedtime. Your urine should be translucent and not have a smell to it. That was free, but again, this is why water is so important.

After water, the second thing is to get rid of table sugar, especially sugary drinks like sodas and even pre-packaged teas. Table sugar has gone through a refining process where it is stripped of its original color and natural properties.

If you must, I suggest you add your own sugar to your drinks so that you have more control, and use more natural sweeteners that are not man-made and don't send your blood sugar out of whack!

There are sweeteners that I feel are better for you and don't do harmful things like weakening your immune system, natural alternatives like monk fruit, dates, stevia or even agave. I recommend adding only a small amount of sweetener to your food and drink so that you don't become addicted or dependent upon it. Again, don't let your mind bully your body.

Lastly, let's get you moving! Below are a few exercise circuits you can use to get you started. Start where you are. Listen to your body. Push yourself to the next level when you are ready. No equipment necessary!

However, it is easy to incorporate everyday items around your house like furniture, a step stool, bottles of water or even cans of soup to add a little weight to any of the arm exercises. A resistance band or dumbbells can be purchased and incorporated during intermediate or advanced workouts if you like, but again not necessary.

Start off with five pounds and when those are too light head up to ten or twelve pounds. With resistance bands, you can also start off light, then increase resistance as you advance in your workouts. Resistance bands are color coded by difficulty. Perform a search online to understand the difference in colors and resistance prior to purchasing.

As you begin your workouts, I recommend you include some praise and worship music to take glorifying God in our bodies all the way home. I promote and live by all of the dynamic duos in health and wellness: Faith and Fitness, Workout and Worship, Diet and Exercise. You see where I'm going with this?

I'm including a few more of my favorite worship songs, ones that I love to work out to. I often have them playing throughout the day or around the house—and sometimes break out in a dance like David did! And guess what! That is a form of exercise too.

Put on a few of your favorite songs. I recommend ones that point to the Father and magnify Him for all He has done and all He is doing! Whoop, Whoop, and get at it! Cut a rug, jump around, have a good time with your Creator and burn some calories while you are at it—not to mention having a little fun too!

I told you God speaks to me through songs! Choose one for each day of the week or one per week for seven weeks or however you see fit. I believe that something supernatural happens when worship God. It shifts the atmosphere. So, try it and let's see that happens!

Great Worship Songs for Working Out

- *Hosanna* – Kirk Franklin
- *Yes, I Will* – Vertical Worship
- *Reckless Love* – Cory Asbury
- *Run to the Father* – Cody Carnes
- *Famous* – Tauryn Wells
- *Give Me Faith* – Elevation Worship
- *Man of Your Word* – Maverick City

Below are a few takeaways from Chapter Eight. You may choose to come back and reflect on these later.

Lessons:

A. Now is the time to just start!

B. Incorporating the three tips, of increased water intake, eliminating table sugar and start moving will make a huge difference that you will see quickly.

C. Worship God at all times, even while working out!

<u>Confessions:</u>

- I commit my works unto You Lord, and my thoughts are established. (Proverbs 16:3).

- I am confident of this very thing, that He who has begun a good work in me will complete it until the day of Jesus Christ. (Philippians 1:6).

- I press toward the goal for the prize of the upward call of God in Christ Jesus. (Philippians 3:14).

- Surely goodness and mercy shall follow me all the days of my life: and I will dwell in the house of the LORD for ever. (Psalm 23:6).

- I wait on the LORD and my strength is renewed; I mount up with wings like eagles, I run and am not weary, I walk and am not faint. (Isaiah 40:31).

- I trust in the LORD, and do good; I dwell in the land, and feed on His faithfulness. (Psalm 37:3).

Prayer:

Father,

I am ready to take the next steps and I invite you along on the journey. I admit, this is a little scary, but I'm committed to living a healthy Kingdom Lifestyle and I'm committed to soaring in my faith and fitness because I am committed to you. Thank you for holding my hand every step of the way. I look forward to seeing You complete the good work that you started in me! In Jesus Name I pray! Amen!

<u>Workouts</u>

Now let's get to the moving part of you soaring in your faith and fitness. Below, are some practical exercises that you can begin to incorporate upon your doctor's approval at various level.

<u>Beginner Workout – 2 Options</u>

Gauge for yourself as to how much physical activity is good to start with. Don't be too hard or too soft on yourself. Listen to your body if you are experiencing pain while doing any exercise and stop immediately. However, continue to push yourself if you feel a little soreness after you have done some movement.

Option 1

Start with a basic walk. You can do this around your neighborhood, the local park or school track. Download an app to your phone, use trackers like fit bit, or a pedometer to see how many steps, pace, calories burned and time it takes for your walk. Use these measures to continue to improve and go to the next level. Sooner or later, you will be jogging—and then running in no time!

Option 2

You will need to use a chair for stability and sitting for these exercises. Stand behind the chair for the first 3 exercises and sit in the chair for the second set of exercises.

Circuit 1

1. 12 leg swings holding the back of the chair—3 Rounds each leg
2. 12 squats holding the back of the chair—3 Rounds
3. 12 marches in place holding the back of the chair—3 Rounds

Circuit 2

1. 12 arm circles, both arms together, backward, then forward sitting in the chair—3 rounds each leg
2. 12 knee drives towards your chest sitting in the chair—3 rounds each leg
3. 12 punches each arm sitting in the chair—3 Rounds

Intermediate Workouts

Joining a local gym and attending a fitness class is always an option. You could also find online virtual programs like those we offer at KPL. If you are unable to attend a class and want to do a few things on your own, try one of the workouts below. I like Circuit Training as well as mixing things up between upper body, lower body, full body and muscle group focus like glutes or chest, for example. I also like simple options where you can use items around your house as I understand not everyone has an in-home gym.

Option 1

Tabata Work out—perform each exercise for 20 seconds and rest for 10 seconds for 8 rounds.

There are 8 exercises, 40 seconds work, 20 seconds rest repeating for 8 rounds. See below:

Tabata:

1. Fast feet twists
2. Elbow to knee
3. Squat and touch
4. In and out crunch
5. Fast feet in and out
6. Plank tap and reach

7. Step up with knee drive and lunge, alternating legs each round

8. Alternating twist and kick

Repeat 8 rounds

Option 2 - Full Body

Crazy Eights—If you are not familiar with any of these exercises, search Google or our YouTube channel to see examples.

1. 8 Jumping jacks
2. 8 Squats
3. 8 Lunges
4. 8 Mountain climbers
5. 8 Triceps dips
6. 8 Bicycle crunches
7. 8 Push ups
8. 8 Burpees

Advanced Workouts

At this point, you may choose to join a gym, or regular exercise program, or hire a personal trainer. However, if you would like to perform some workouts on your own, below are a couple of options.

Option 1 - Full Body

There are 6 exercises in total, which make up one round. Perform for 1 minute each with a 30-45 second rest in between, then repeat for 4-5 rounds.

Circuit

1. Predator jack 1 minute
2. Back extension to push up 1 minute
3. Sprinters crunch 1 minute
4. Up and down or kneeling to squat 1 minute
5. Triceps dip with knee drive 1 minute
6. Double elbow to knee crunch 1 minute

30-45 sec rest then repeat
    7.

Option 2 - Core Strength

5 exercises for our killer core workout. A strong core is very important, so perform each exercise for 1 minute. If that is too much, reduce to 30-45 seconds and build up to 1 minute. This makes up one round. Rest for 30-45 seconds in between rounds. Repeat for 4-5 rounds.

Circuit

1. Bear hold to knee drop 1 minute
2. Plank wall-ups 1 minute
3. Dead bug 1 minute
4. Plank jack to alternating knee drive 1 minute
5. Reverse plank to alternating kick 1 minute

30-45 sec rest then repeat x 4

CLOSING

If you are reading this book, chances are you are a believer in Jesus Christ. However, if you are not or want to make a rededication to Him, please pray the following prayer.

Dear Heavenly Father! I acknowledge that I am a sinner and I need you to save me. I know that I have lived my life in reliance on myself instead of you. So now, I invite you into my heart as my Lord and my Savior. I ask you to cleanse me and make me new. I no longer want to live on my terms so I confess with my mouth and believe in my heart that Christ Jesus died on the cross to save me. And from this day forward I ask you to never leave me. In Jesus Name I pray! Amen.

ABOUT THE AUTHOR

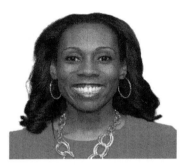 April Griffith is an inspirational speaker, mindset strategist and fitness coach. After years of working in Higher Education and Corporate America at one of the largest financial institutions in the world, April realized that through her expanded volunteer work with several internal groups, she had helped shape the lives of many professionals. This sparked a passion inside and caused her to launch into an entrepreneurial career and birth Kingdom Power Living with the mission of changing lives one temple at a time!

In April's mindset, combined with health and wellness work, she helps her clients lose weight by leaning on their faith. April challenges her clients to invite God in on the journey to change both the inside and outside, leading to lasting change and the kingdom lifestyle they deserve. She is a certified fitness trainer with a vision to get the Body of Christ moving and making sound health choices! She is also the creator of both the *3 With Me, 3 Minutes of Exercise in 3 Days* and *Food For Thought, 'Cleaning up Your Diet so You Won't Need One' Challenges*.

A sought-after emcee, moderator, panelist and speaker, April has led thought provoking interviews with brilliant minds such as Mellody Hobson and Maria Pinto, and been opening emcee for Nick Cannon's Chicago Girls and Boys Club Entrepreneur Competition.

April is active in her church, where she has mentored dozens of college students over the years and currently mentors elementary school kids with the Wood Family Foundation. She has served on a number of steering and leadership committees around diversity and women's issues, including the board for the *Chicago Chapter National Black MBA Association, Inc.* and is a previous recipient of *Diversity MBA's 100 Under 50 Emerging Leaders*.

April holds a Bachelor of Science in Broadcast Communication from Northwest Missouri State University, and a Master of Science in Marketing Communication from IIT's Stuart School of Business, where she was Valedictorian and Class Speaker. She is a native of Chicago, a sports enthusiast, and avid volunteer with organizations such as *Junior Achievement Chicago, One Million Degrees, Habitat Chicago, Big Shoulders and Chicago Cares*.

Contact April Griffith For Fitness

www.kingdompowerliving.com

hello@kingdompowerliving.com

Social Media: @kingdompowerliving

Mail Correspondence

17 E. Monroe, #187

Chicago, IL 60603

Made in the USA
Monee, IL
04 May 2021